The Holistic Soul

By Asante Bradford

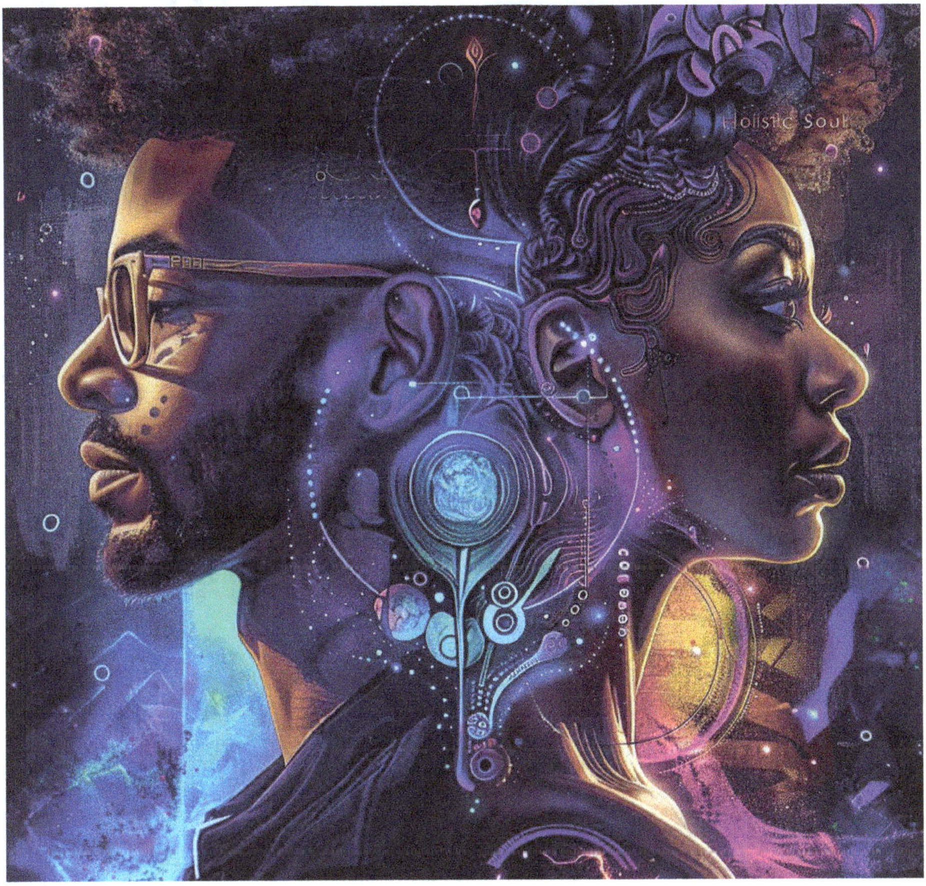

Wellness Practices Rooted in Black Tradition

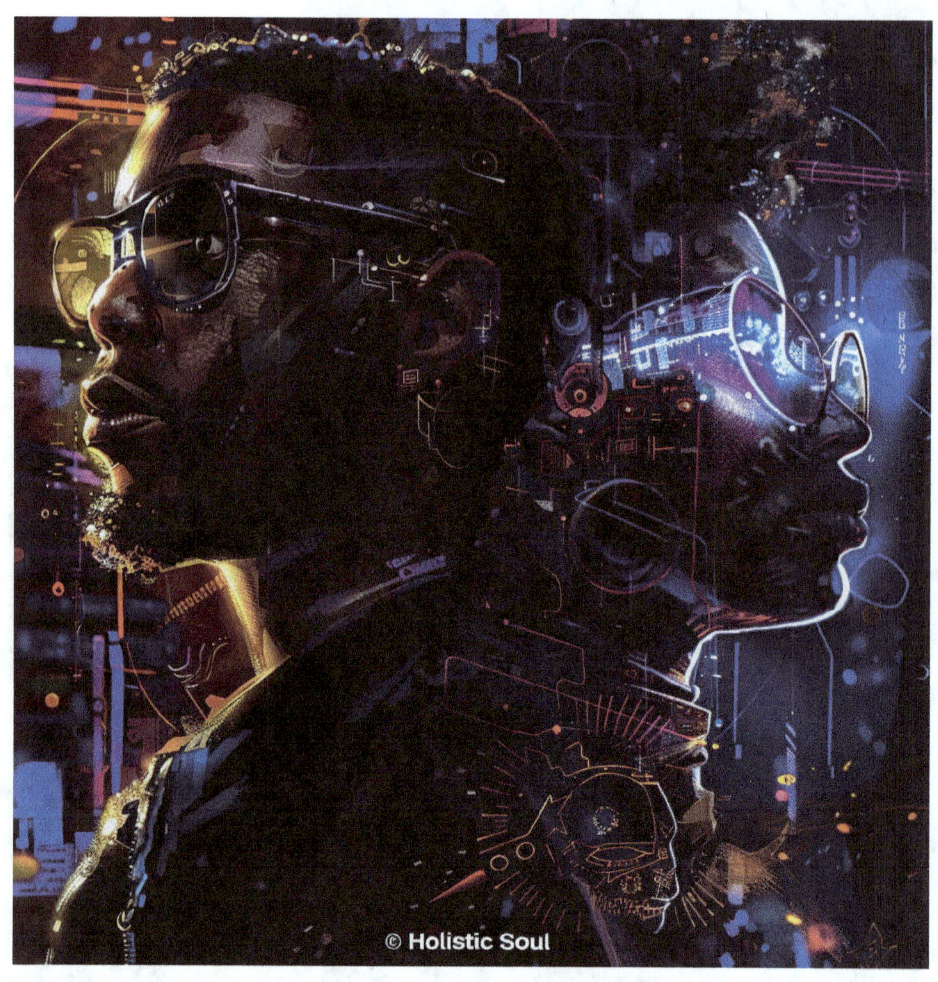
© Holistic Soul

The Holistic Soul: Wellness Practices Rooted in Black Tradition

Written by and Cover Design - Asante Bradford

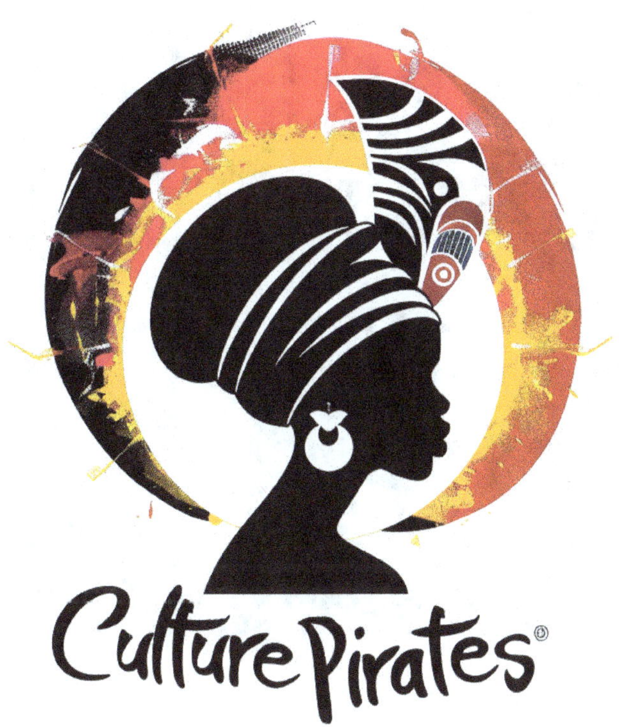

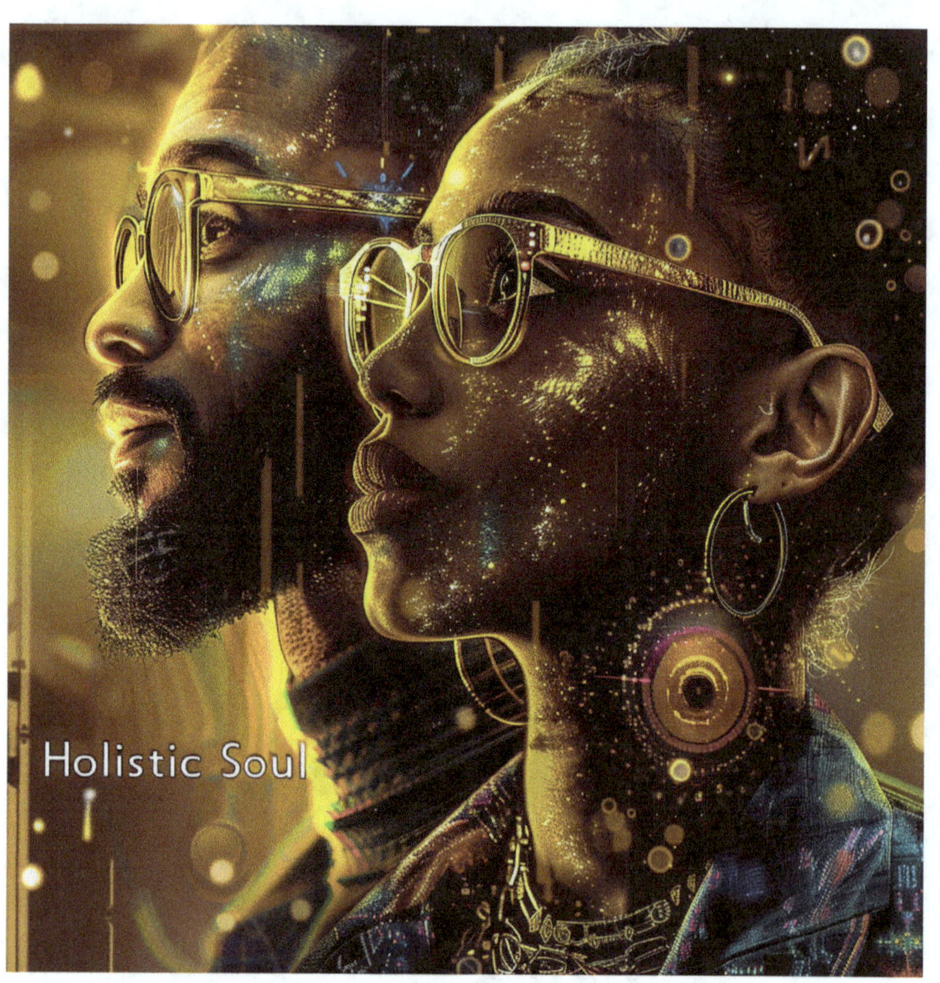
Holistic Soul

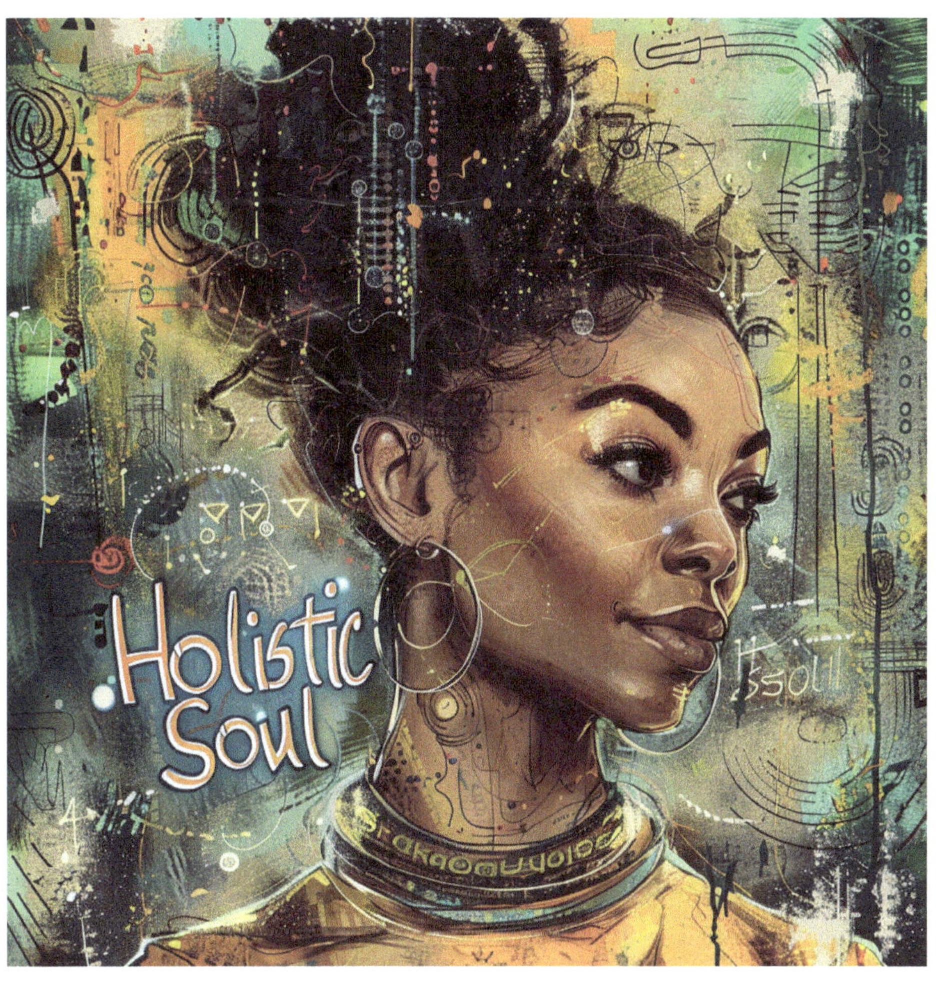

Holistic
Soul

Preface

"The Holistic Soul: Wellness Practices Rooted in Black Tradition" is a groundbreaking exploration of holistic health approaches that blend the wisdom of African and African American cultural practices with modern scientific understanding. In a world where health disparities continue to affect Black communities disproportionately, this book offers a return to ancestral knowledge as a pathway to wellness.

From the bustling markets of West Africa to the community gardens of urban America, Black cultures have long held secrets to vibrant health and longevity. This book uncovers these treasures, presenting them in a context that is both accessible and applicable to contemporary life. We delve into traditional nutritional practices, healing rituals, movement as medicine, and the profound connection between spirituality and physical well-being.

"The Holistic Soul" is not just a health guide; it's a celebration of Black resilience and ingenuity. It honors the generations who preserved these practices through centuries of adversity, and it empowers readers to reclaim their health heritage.

Whether you're looking to reconnect with your roots or seeking alternative approaches to wellness, this book offers a rich tapestry of knowledge that bridges past and present.

As we navigate the complexities of modern health challenges, "The Holistic Soul" provides a roadmap back to balance, rooted in the strength of Black tradition and illuminated by the light of current medical knowledge. Join us on this journey of discovery, healing, and empowerment.

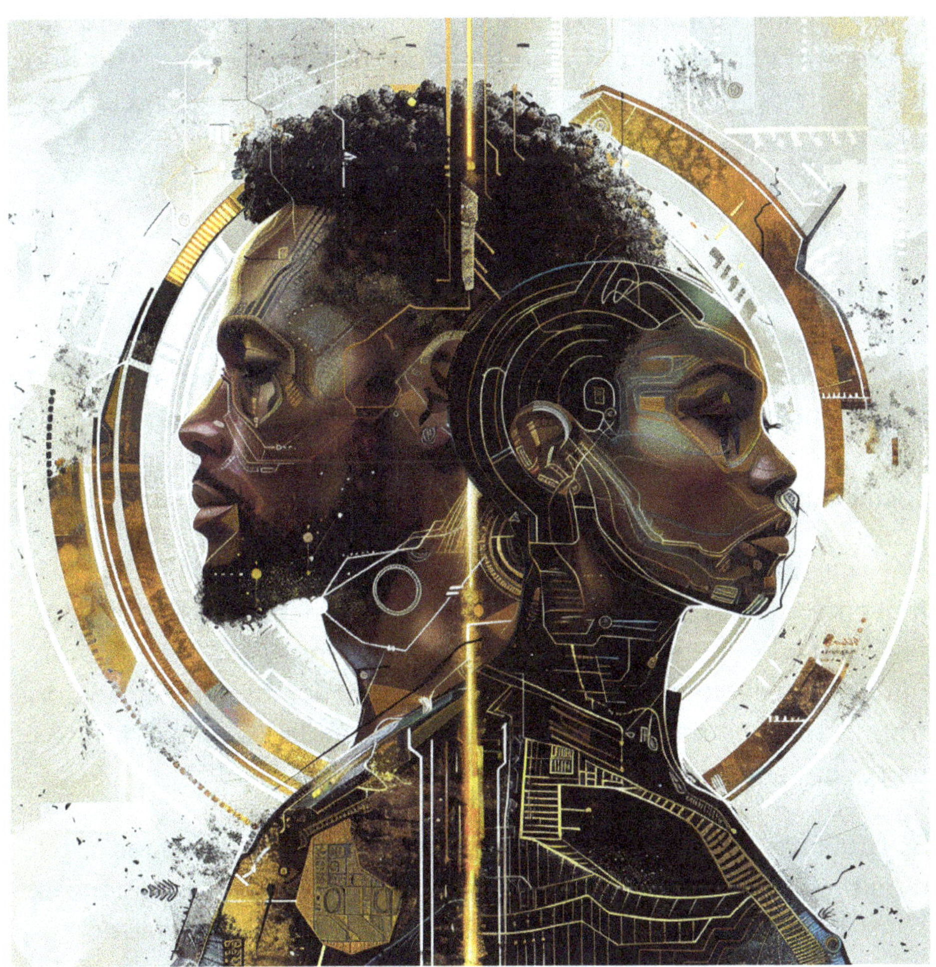

Forward

"The Holistic Soul: Wellness Practices Rooted in Black Tradition" offers a comprehensive exploration of health and wellness through the lens of African and African American cultural wisdom. This book bridges the gap between ancestral practices and modern science, providing readers with practical strategies for achieving holistic well-being.

The journey begins with a deep dive into traditional African nutrition, examining how ancestral diets can be adapted to meet contemporary health needs. We explore the integration of superfoods into soul food recipes, maintaining cultural flavors while enhancing nutritional value. The book then moves beyond the plate, discussing the healing power of community and the importance of social connections in maintaining mental and emotional health.

Physical wellness is addressed through the lens of traditional movement practices, from ritual dances to practical exercises that can be incorporated into modern lifestyles. The wisdom of natural remedies is explored, with a careful examination of herbal traditions from Africa and the African diaspora, and guidance on how these can complement modern medical approaches.

Spirituality's role in wellness is a key focus, exploring how faith, meditation, and mindfulness practices rooted in Black traditions can contribute to overall health. The book concludes with a holistic approach to self-care, offering rituals and practices that nurture both body and soul.

Throughout, "The Holistic Soul" emphasizes the importance of reclaiming and honoring Black health traditions while adapting them to address current health challenges. It serves as both a practical guide and a cultural celebration, empowering readers to take control of their health journey with tools deeply rooted in their heritage.

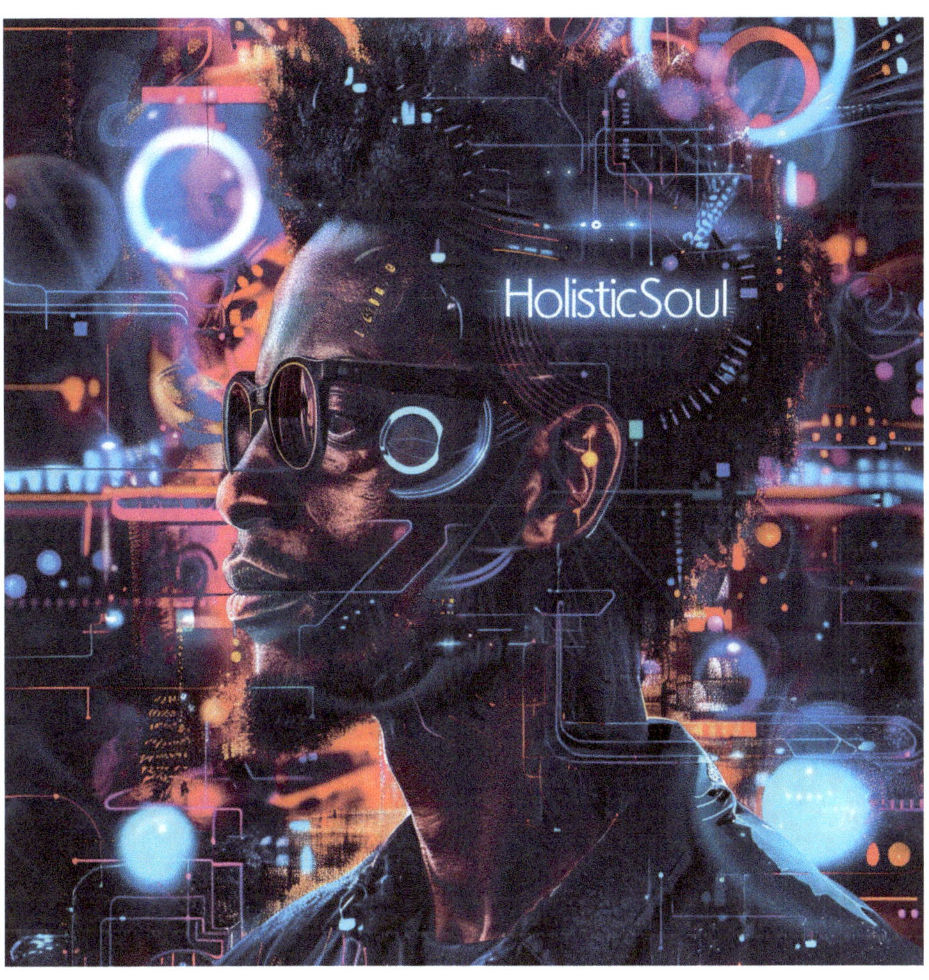
HolisticSoul

Introduction

"The Holistic Soul: Wellness Practices Rooted in Black Tradition" is a transformative guide that bridges the wisdom of African and African American healing traditions with contemporary health science.

This book offers a holistic approach to wellness that speaks directly to the Black experience, addressing the unique health challenges faced by our communities while celebrating the rich cultural heritage that has sustained us for generations.

In these pages, you will embark on a journey of discovery and empowerment. We delve into the heart of Black wellness traditions, exploring:

• The power of nutrition through a reimagining of soul food, blending traditional flavors with modern superfoods

• The healing potential of movement, from ancestral dances to adaptable exercise routines

• The strength found in community and its impact on mental and emotional well-being

• The wisdom of natural remedies and herbal traditions passed down through generations

• The profound connection between spirituality and physical health

• Holistic self-care practices that nourish both body and soul

This book is not just a collection of health tips; it's a roadmap to reclaiming your wellness heritage. It acknowledges the historical and ongoing health disparities affecting Black communities while offering practical, culturally resonant solutions. By interweaving personal stories, historical context, and cutting-edge research,

"The Holistic Soul" provides a comprehensive framework for achieving optimal health that honors our past while embracing our future.

Whether you're looking to address specific health concerns, reconnect with your cultural roots, or simply enhance your overall well-being, this book offers invaluable insights and actionable strategies.

It's an invitation to rediscover the healer within you and to tap into the collective wisdom of our ancestors.

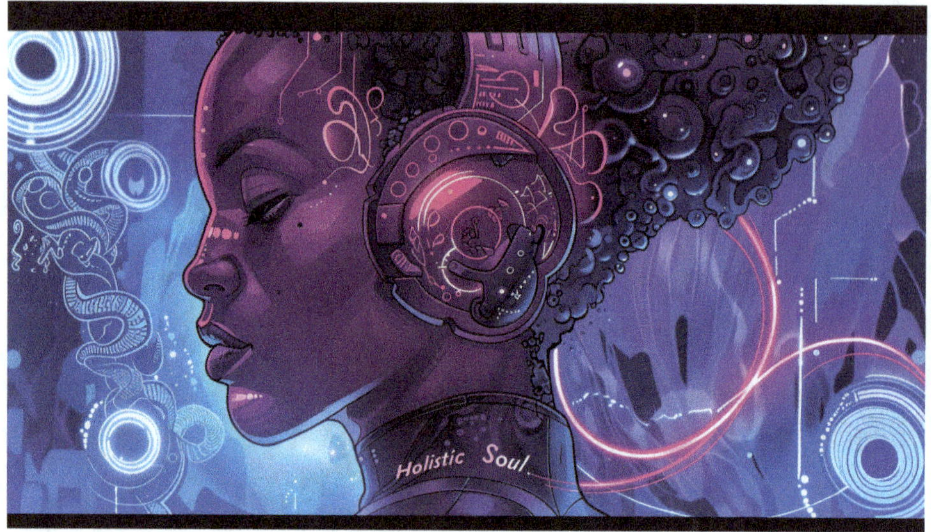

As you journey through these pages, prepare to be inspired, challenged, and ultimately empowered.

"The Holistic Soul" is more than a wellness guide—it's a celebration of Black resilience, a testament to our innovative spirit, and a powerful tool for personal and community transformation.

Welcome to a new chapter in your health journey, one that's deeply rooted in the strength of Black tradition.

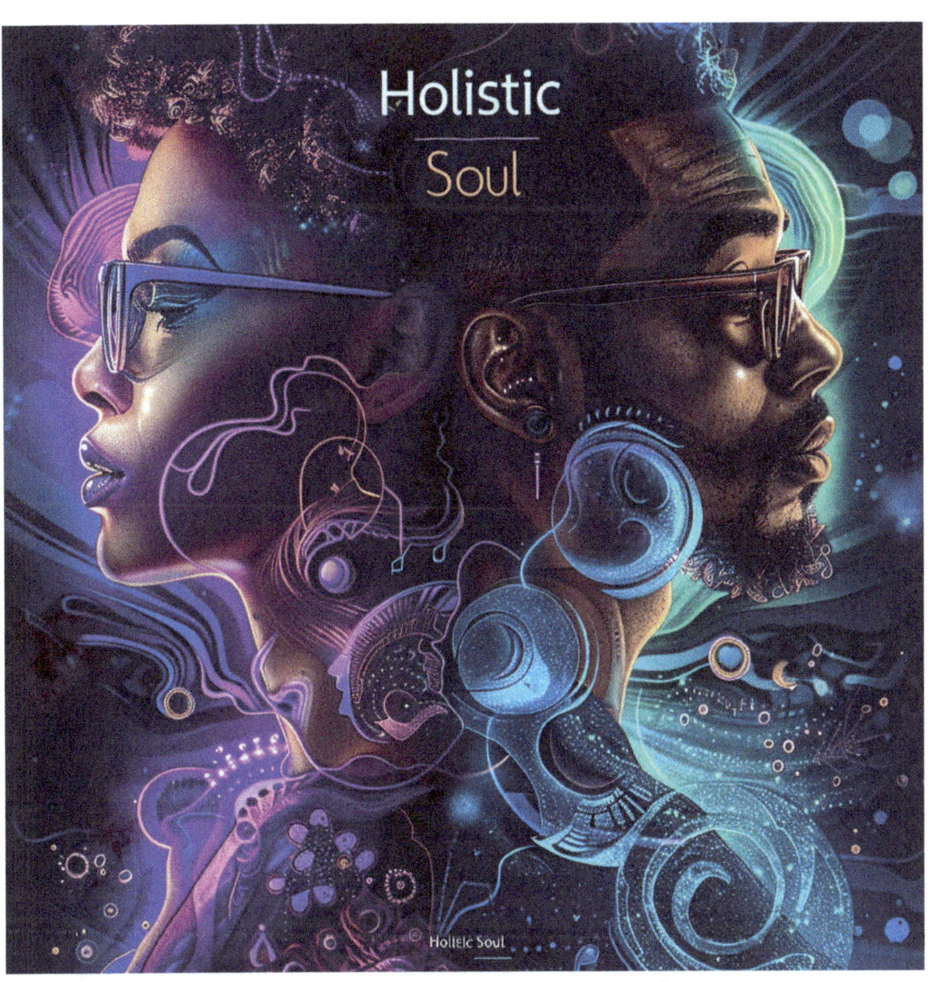

Holistic
Soul
Holleic Soul

FROM THE AUTHOR

As the author of "The Holistic Soul: Wellness Practices Rooted in Black Tradition," I embarked on this project with a profound sense of purpose and personal connection. My journey to write this book began with a simple question: How can we, as Black individuals, reclaim our health while honoring our rich cultural heritage?

Growing up, I witnessed the dichotomy between the vibrant, communal aspects of our food culture and the health challenges that plagued many in our community. I saw elders who held vast knowledge of natural remedies, yet struggled with chronic diseases. I experienced the spiritual strength that uplifted us through adversity, but also saw how stress and trauma impacted our collective well-being.

This book is born out of a desire to bridge these gaps – to harness the wisdom of our ancestors and align it with modern health science. It's a labor of love, fueled by countless hours of research, interviews with community elders, health practitioners, and cultural experts, as well as my own experiences in exploring and applying these practices.

Writing "The Holistic Soul" has been a deeply transformative experience. It has reinforced my belief in the power of our traditions and the resilience of our community. But more importantly, it has filled me with hope. Hope that by reconnecting with our roots and adapting ancient wisdom to modern life, we can address the health disparities that have long affected our community.

This book is not just a guide; it's a call to action. It's an invitation to embark on a journey of self-discovery, to reclaim our narrative around health and wellness. It challenges us to see beyond the limitations often imposed on us and to recognize the healer within each of us.

My vision for "The Holistic Soul" is that it will spark a movement – a return to holistic, culturally affirming health practices that can be passed down to future generations. I hope it empowers readers to take control of their health journey, to question, to explore, and to find joy in the process of nurturing their body, mind, and spirit.

As you read this book, I encourage you to approach it with an open heart and mind. Try the practices, adapt them to your life, and share them with your community. Remember, our ancestors' wisdom has sustained us through centuries of challenges. By honoring and evolving these traditions, we can forge a healthier, more vibrant future for ourselves and for generations to come.

Warmly,

Asante Bradford

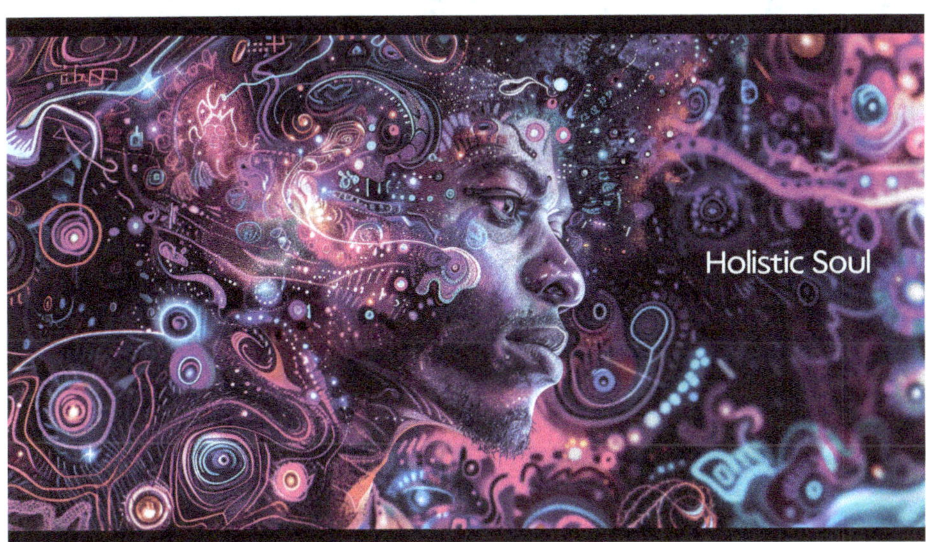

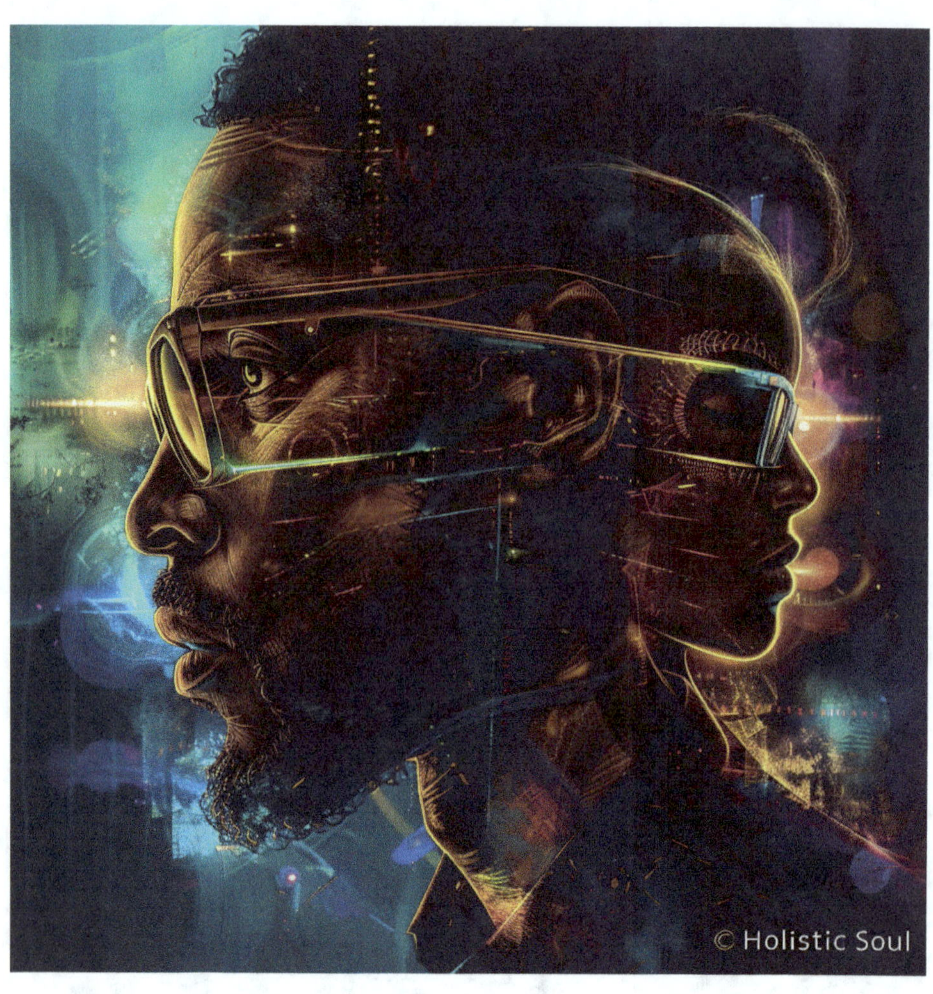
© Holistic Soul

Table of Contents

Chapter Descriptions:

1. Ancestral Nutrition: Reclaiming Our Culinary Heritage This chapter explores the rich tapestry of African and African American culinary traditions, examining how traditional diets supported health and vitality. It delves into the nutritional wisdom of our ancestors and offers practical ways to adapt soul food recipes for optimal health. Readers will learn about indigenous African superfoods, the balance of flavors and nutrients in traditional meals, and how to incorporate these principles into modern cooking.
2. The Healing Power of Community This chapter examines the crucial role that community plays in Black wellness traditions. It explores how social connections, family structures, and communal practices have historically contributed to resilience and health in Black communities.
3. Movement as Medicine: Traditional Dance and Exercise This chapter focuses on the importance of physical activity in Black wellness traditions, with a particular emphasis on dance and rhythmic movement. It explores the cultural and spiritual significance of traditional African and African American dances, their health benefits, and how they can be adapted for modern fitness routines. The chapter also covers other forms of traditional exercise and physical practices, offering readers practical ways to incorporate these movements into their daily lives for improved physical and mental health.

4. Natural Remedies and Herbal Wisdom This chapter delves into the rich tradition of herbal medicine in Black cultures, from African healing practices to remedies developed during slavery and beyond. It provides an overview of common herbs used in Black traditional medicine, their purported benefits, and how to use them safely alongside modern medical practices. The chapter also explores the historical context of these remedies and how this knowledge has been preserved and passed down through generations.

5. The Spirituality of Wellness This chapter examines the intrinsic connection between spirituality and health in Black traditions. It explores various spiritual practices, including prayer, meditation, and rituals, and their impact on mental, emotional, and physical well-being. The chapter discusses how to integrate spiritual practices into daily life for stress reduction, emotional healing, and overall wellness. It also addresses the role of faith communities in supporting health and how to navigate the intersection of spirituality and modern healthcare.

6. Holistic Self-Care: Nurturing the Black Body and Mind The final chapter brings together all elements of Black wellness traditions into a comprehensive approach to self-care. It offers practical strategies for developing a personalized wellness routine that honors cultural heritage while addressing individual health needs. Topics include stress management techniques rooted in Black traditions, beauty and skincare practices, sleep hygiene informed by ancestral wisdom, and methods for maintaining emotional well-being. The chapter emphasizes the importance of self-love and self-acceptance as fundamental aspects of Black wellness.

THE HOLISTIC SOUL

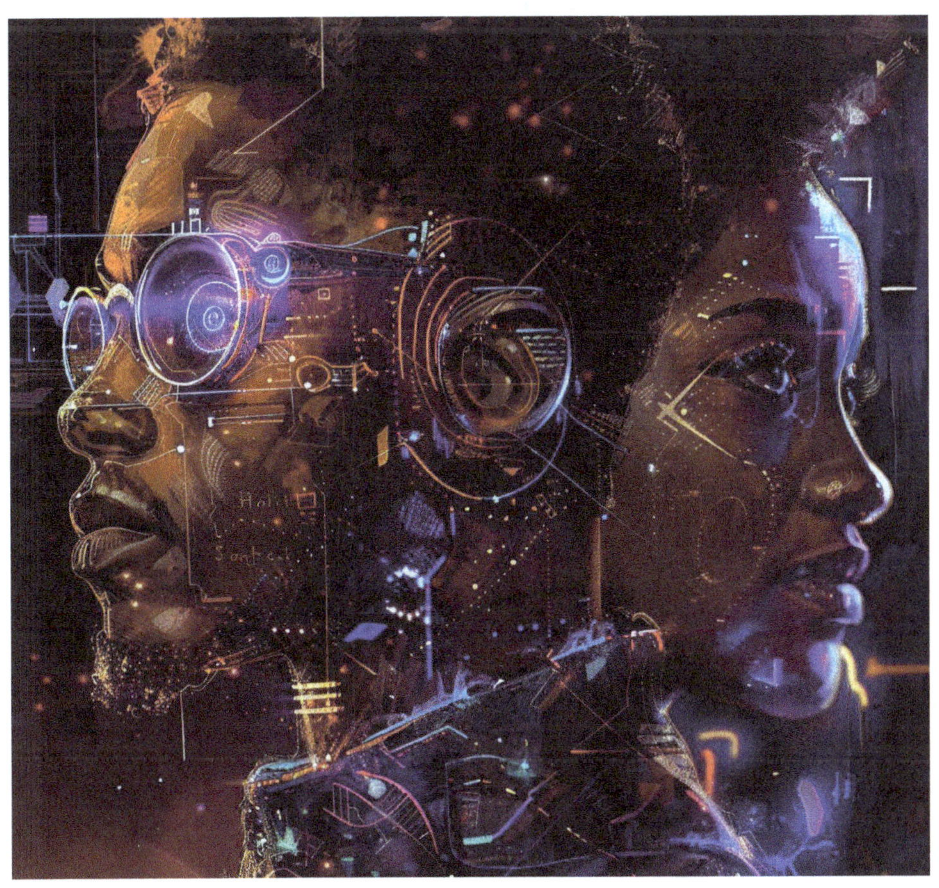

Wellness Practices Rooted in Black Tradition

1

Soul food has long been a cornerstone of Black culinary tradition, celebrated for its rich flavors and cultural significance. However, as our understanding of nutrition and health has evolved, there has been a growing recognition of the need to adapt traditional recipes to meet modern dietary needs. This shift has given rise to the concept of incorporating superfoods into the Black diet, blending the best of ancestral wisdom with contemporary nutritional science.

Traditional African diets are characterized by their emphasis on whole foods, plant-based ingredients, and a balance of macronutrients. Staples such as leafy greens, legumes, and whole grains form the foundation of these diets, providing a wealth of essential vitamins, minerals, and fiber. These nutrient-dense foods not only support overall health but also have been linked to a reduced risk of chronic diseases such as heart disease, diabetes, and obesity.

One of the key principles of adapting soul food recipes for modern nutritional needs is to focus on quality ingredients and mindful cooking techniques. By choosing fresh, locally sourced produce and minimizing the use of processed foods high in added sugars and unhealthy fats, we can preserve the essence of soul food while enhancing its health benefits. For example, swapping out traditional ingredients like lard and excessive amounts of salt for healthier alternatives like olive oil and herbs can significantly improve the nutritional profile of classic dishes.

Incorporating indigenous African superfoods into daily meals is another way to elevate the nutritional value of traditional recipes. Foods like moringa, baobab, fonio, and sorghum are nutrient powerhouses, packed with antioxidants, vitamins, and minerals that support immune function, digestion, and overall vitality.

These superfoods not only add depth of flavor and texture to dishes but also contribute to a more diverse and nutrient-rich diet.

By embracing the concept of From Soul Food to Superfoods, we are not only honoring our culinary heritage but also investing in our health and well-being for generations to come. This approach encourages us to celebrate the flavors and traditions of soul food while also recognizing the importance of nourishing our bodies with wholesome, nutrient-dense foods. Through a thoughtful blend of ancestral wisdom and modern nutritional science, we can create a vibrant and sustainable food culture that promotes health, vitality, and connection to our roots.

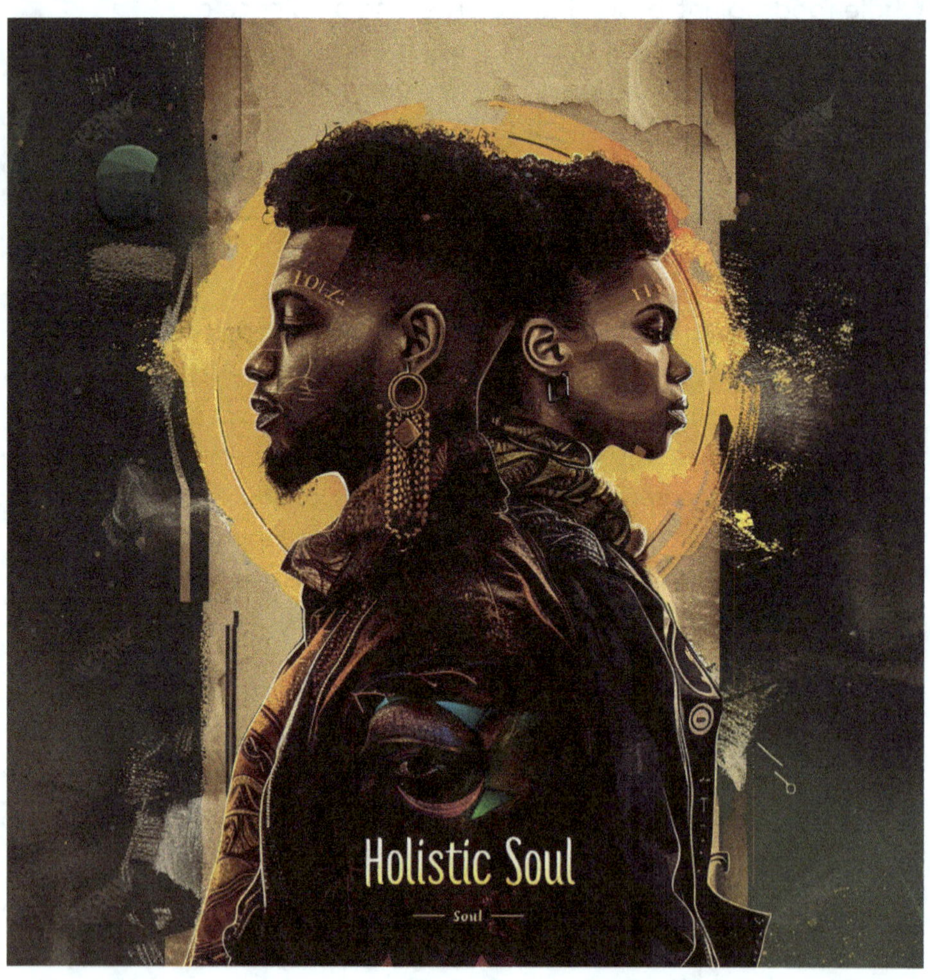

1.2: Traditional African diets and their health benefits

Traditional African diets are a reflection of centuries-old culinary practices that have been passed down through generations. These diets are not only flavorful and rich in cultural significance but also offer a range of health benefits that are increasingly being recognized and appreciated in modern times.

One of the key principles of traditional African diets is their emphasis on whole, minimally processed foods. These diets typically consist of a variety of fruits, vegetables, whole grains, legumes, nuts, seeds, and lean proteins such as fish and poultry.

This diverse array of nutrient-dense foods provides a wide range of essential vitamins, minerals, and antioxidants that support overall health and well-being.

Traditional African diets are also known for their reliance on plant-based foods. Vegetables like okra, collard greens, sweet potatoes, and yams are staples in many traditional African cuisines.

 These vegetables are not only rich in fiber and essential nutrients but also have been linked to a reduced risk of chronic diseases such as heart disease, diabetes, and certain types of cancer.

Another hallmark of traditional African diets is the use of whole grains such as sorghum, millet, and teff. These grains are rich in fiber, vitamins, and minerals and have a lower glycemic index compared to refined grains, which can help regulate blood sugar levels and reduce the risk of diabetes and obesity.

Legumes such as black-eyed peas, lentils, and chickpeas are also commonly included in traditional African diets. These plant-based proteins are not only a great source of essential amino acids but also contain fiber, iron, and other important nutrients that support muscle health, cardiovascular health, and overall well-being.

Incorporating traditional African dietary practices into modern nutrition can offer a range of health benefits. Research has shown that adherence to a traditional African diet can help lower the risk of chronic diseases such as obesity, diabetes, and cardiovascular disease.

The emphasis on whole, minimally processed foods, plant-based ingredients, and nutrient-dense staples makes traditional African diets a valuable source of inspiration for individuals looking to improve their overall health and well-being.

Overall, traditional African diets offer a holistic approach to nutrition that focuses on nourishing the body with wholesome, nutrient-rich foods that support optimal health and vitality.

By embracing the principles of ancestral nutrition and reclaiming the culinary heritage of traditional African diets, individuals can not only enjoy delicious and culturally significant meals but also promote long-term health and well-being.

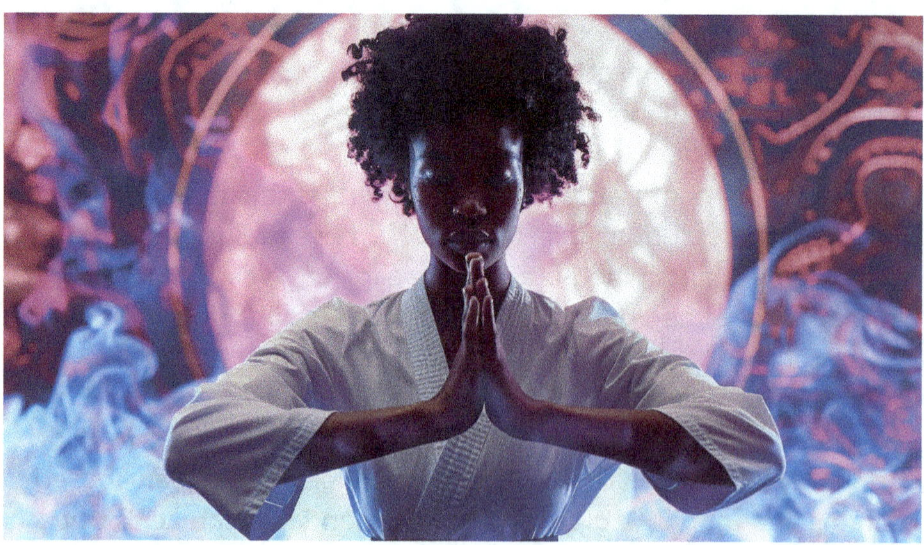

1.3: Adapting soul food recipes for modern nutritional needs

Soul food has long been a beloved culinary tradition within the Black community, rooted in history and culture. However, traditional soul food dishes are often laden with ingredients high in fats, sugars, and sodium, which can contribute to health issues such as heart disease, diabetes, and obesity.

In light of these concerns, there is a growing movement to adapt soul food recipes to meet modern nutritional needs while still honoring the rich flavors and traditions of this cuisine.

One approach to adapting soul food recipes is to focus on ingredient substitutions. For example, instead of using lard or bacon fat for cooking, healthier options like olive oil or avocado oil can be used. Switching out refined white flour for whole grain flours or alternative flours such as almond or coconut can increase the fiber content and reduce the glycemic load of dishes.

Similarly, replacing traditional white sugar with natural sweeteners like honey, maple syrup, or dates can help lower the overall sugar content of recipes.

Another key aspect of adapting soul food recipes for modern nutritional needs is to increase the emphasis on plant-based ingredients. By incorporating more fruits, vegetables, whole grains, legumes, and nuts into dishes, it is possible to boost the fiber, vitamins, minerals, and antioxidants in the meal while reducing the reliance on animal products that are often high in saturated fats.

For example, adding collard greens, sweet potatoes, okra, and black-eyed peas to traditional dishes can increase the nutrient density and provide a wider range of health benefits.

 Furthermore, portion control and mindful eating play a crucial role in adapting soul food recipes for modern nutritional needs.

By being mindful of serving sizes and listening to hunger cues, individuals can enjoy soul food dishes in a balanced and healthful way.

Additionally, incorporating cooking techniques such as baking, grilling, steaming, or sautéing instead of deep-frying can help reduce the overall calorie and fat content of meals.

In addition to ingredient substitutions and focusing on plant-based ingredients, incorporating herbs, spices, and seasonings can enhance the flavor profiles of adapted soul food recipes without compromising on taste.

By using herbs like thyme, oregano, basil, and spices like cumin, chili powder, and turmeric, it is possible to create delicious and satisfying meals that are also nutritious and supportive of overall health.

By making mindful ingredient choices, emphasizing plant-based ingredients, practicing portion control, and using herbs and spices creatively, it is possible to enjoy the flavors of soul food while promoting optimal health and wellbeing.

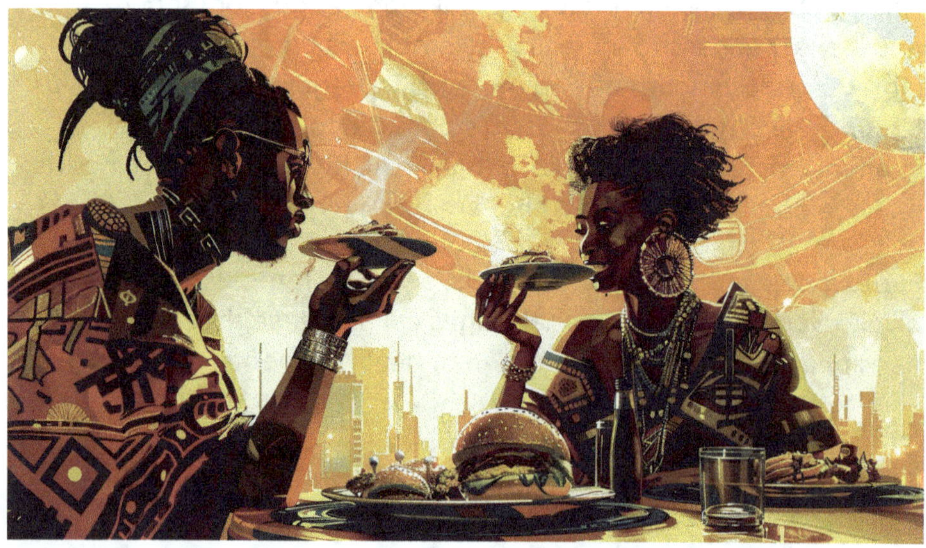

1.4: Incorporating indigenous African superfoods into daily meals

Incorporating indigenous African superfoods into daily meals is a powerful way to connect with one's ancestral roots while also reaping the nutritional benefits of these nutrient-dense foods.

Traditional African diets are rich in a variety of superfoods that have been used for generations to promote health and vitality. By reintroducing these foods into our modern diets, we can not only improve our physical health but also honor the culinary heritage of our ancestors.

One of the key components of traditional African diets is the use of whole, unprocessed foods that are rich in nutrients. Superfoods like moringa, baobab, fonio, and tigernuts are staples in many African cuisines and offer a wide range of health benefits.

Moringa, for example, is a nutrient powerhouse that is high in vitamins, minerals, and antioxidants. It has been used for centuries in African traditional medicine to boost immunity and promote overall health.

Baobab fruit is another superfood that is native to Africa and is known for its high vitamin C content and antioxidant properties. Baobab powder can be easily incorporated into smoothies, baked goods, and other dishes to add a tangy flavor and a nutritional boost.

Fonio is a type of ancient grain that is gluten-free and packed with essential nutrients like iron, zinc, and magnesium. It is a versatile ingredient that can be used in place of rice or couscous in traditional African dishes or as a base for salads and grain bowls.

Tigernuts are not actually nuts but small root vegetables that are rich in fiber, vitamins, and minerals. They can be eaten raw as a snack, ground into flour for baking, or used to make dairy-free tigernut milk.

Incorporating these indigenous African superfoods into daily meals can be as simple as adding them to smoothies, salads, soups, stews, or using them as toppings for yogurt or oatmeal. By diversifying our diet with these nutrient-dense foods, we can enhance our overall health and well-being.

Furthermore, by supporting the cultivation and consumption of indigenous African superfoods, we can also contribute to the preservation of traditional agricultural practices and biodiversity. Many of these superfoods are grown using sustainable farming methods that have been passed down through generations, making them not only beneficial for our health but also for the planet.

By embracing these traditional ingredients, we can reconnect with our roots and experience the health benefits that come from eating a diverse and culturally rich diet.

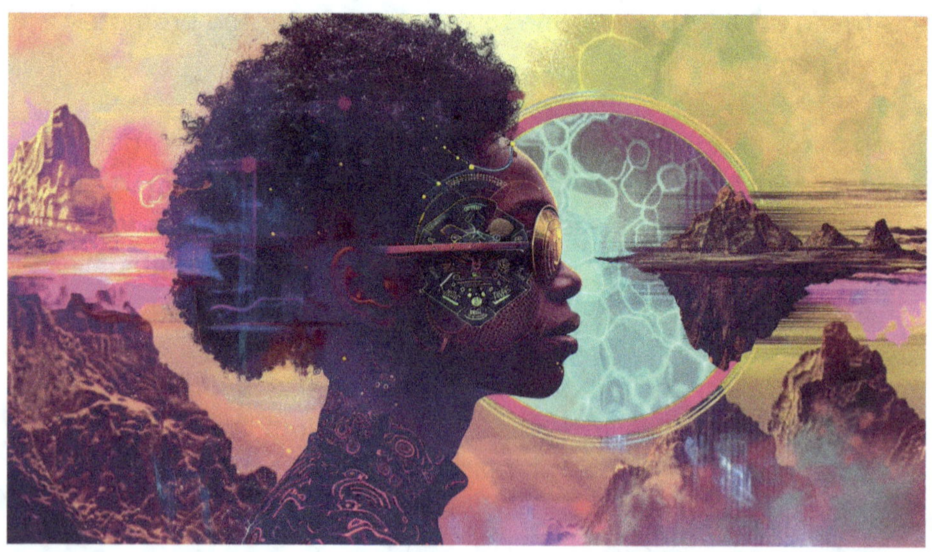

2

Collective Wellness in the Black Experience

In the rich tapestry of Black cultural traditions, the concept of collective wellness plays a vital role in fostering health and healing within communities. Rooted in a history of resilience and interconnectedness, the Black experience in America has long been shaped by the strength and support found within extended family networks and tight-knit communities.

This collective approach to wellness goes beyond individual self-care practices to encompass a holistic view of health that values communal support, shared experiences, and a sense of belonging.

At the heart of collective wellness in the Black experience is the role of extended family and community in promoting mental health and overall well-being. In many Black cultures, the concept of "it takes a village" is deeply ingrained, emphasizing the importance of community support in times of joy and adversity alike.

Extended family members, neighbors, and friends often come together to provide emotional support, practical assistance, and a sense of belonging that nurtures individuals' mental health and resilience.

While traditional communal healing practices have been passed down through generations, modern adaptations have also emerged to meet the evolving needs of Black communities. From support groups and therapy circles to online forums and virtual gatherings, new avenues for collective healing and wellness have been created to address contemporary challenges such as systemic racism, social inequality, and mental health stigma. These spaces provide opportunities for individuals to share their experiences, seek guidance from peers, and access resources that promote mental well-being in a culturally affirming way.

Building and leveraging support networks is essential for fostering collective wellness in the Black experience. By cultivating relationships with trusted community members, mental health professionals, spiritual leaders, and other sources of support, individuals can create a safety net that helps them navigate life's challenges with resilience and strength.

Support networks can take many forms, from informal gatherings and social events to structured programs and organizations that provide resources for mental health education, advocacy, and support services.

In conclusion, collective wellness in the Black experience is a powerful force that draws strength from the interconnectedness of communities, the wisdom of ancestors, and the resilience of individuals who come together in solidarity and compassion.

By embracing the role of extended family and community support, adapting communal healing practices to modern contexts, and building strong support networks, Black individuals can cultivate a culture of wellness that honors their heritage, promotes mental health, and fosters resilience in the face of adversity.

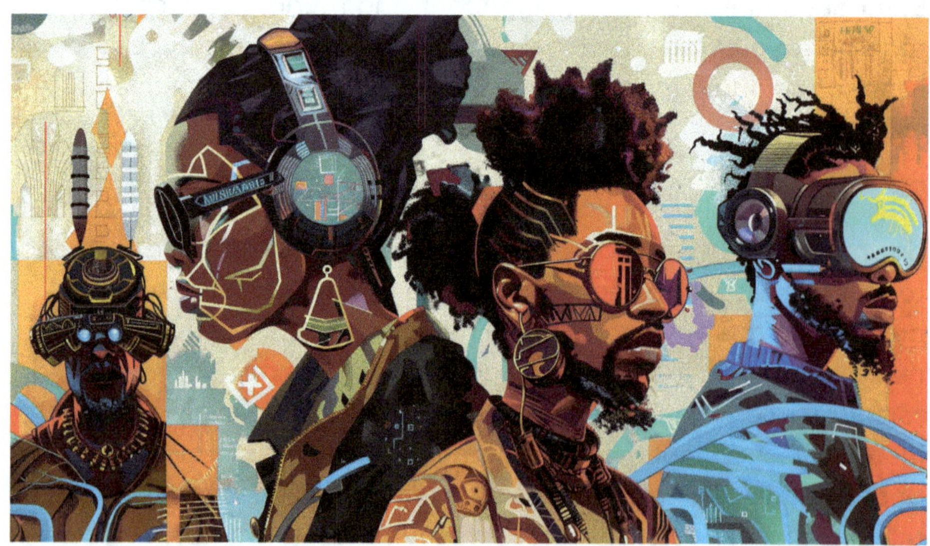

2.2: The role of extended family and community in mental health

The role of extended family and community in mental health is a fundamental aspect of wellness within the Black experience. In many African and African American cultures, the concept of community is deeply ingrained and plays a vital role in supporting individuals' mental health and overall well-being.

Extended family and community serve as pillars of strength and support in navigating life's challenges and triumphs. The communal bond fosters a sense of belonging, connection, and solidarity that can be particularly beneficial in addressing mental health issues. In traditional African societies, the extended family structure extends beyond biological relatives to include a network of individuals who provide emotional, social, and practical support.

Within the Black community, the extended family and community often serve as a source of resilience and empowerment, especially in the face of historical and systemic adversity.

The collective wisdom and shared experiences within these networks offer a sense of shared identity and understanding that can help individuals cope with stress, trauma, and mental health disorders.

Modern adaptations of communal healing practices have emerged as a response to the unique mental health needs of Black individuals. Support groups, community therapy sessions, and culturally relevant counseling services have been developed to provide a safe space for individuals to share their experiences and receive guidance from peers and professionals who understand their cultural background.

Building and leveraging support networks for overall well-being is essential in promoting mental health within the Black community.

By fostering a sense of belonging and collective responsibility, extended family and community members can create a supportive environment where individuals feel valued, respected, and understood.

Community engagement and participation in cultural traditions and celebrations can also contribute to mental well-being by fostering a sense of pride, connection, and cultural continuity.

Traditional practices such as storytelling, music, dance, and art can serve as therapeutic outlets for self-expression, healing, and personal growth.

By fostering strong social connections, offering emotional support, and providing a sense of belonging, these networks play a crucial role in addressing mental health issues and promoting resilience, empowerment, and healing.

Embracing and nurturing these communal bonds can be a powerful tool in promoting mental wellness and enhancing overall quality of life.

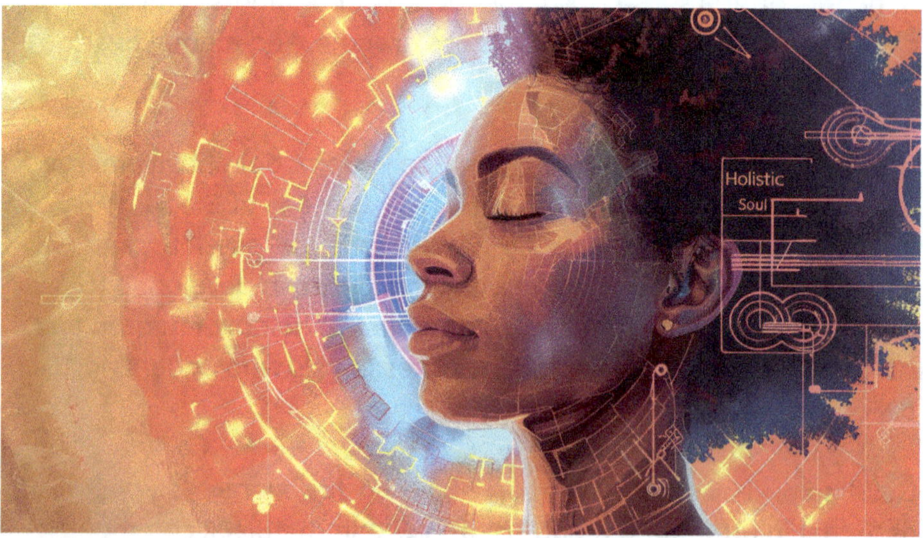

2.3: Modern adaptations of communal healing practices

Modern adaptations of communal healing practices draw from the rich history of collective wellness in the Black experience, emphasizing the importance of extended family and community support in promoting mental health and overall wellbeing.

This section explores how traditional communal healing practices have evolved to address contemporary challenges and needs within the African and African American communities.

In the traditional African context, communal healing practices have long been central to maintaining the health and vitality of individuals within the community. The role of extended family and community support systems is paramount, providing a sense of belonging, connection, and shared responsibility for the wellbeing of all members.

This collective approach to healing recognizes the interdependence of individuals and the power of community in fostering resilience and wellness.

In modern times, the concept of communal healing has been adapted to address the unique stressors and barriers faced by Black individuals and communities. Recognizing the impact of systemic racism, social inequities, and historical trauma on mental health, contemporary communal healing practices aim to create safe spaces for healing, empowerment, and solidarity.

One way in which communal healing practices have been modernized is through the creation of support networks and community-based organizations that offer culturally relevant mental health services and resources. These initiatives provide avenues for individuals to connect with others who share similar experiences and challenges, fostering a sense of community and understanding that is vital for healing and resilience.

Additionally, modern adaptations of communal healing practices often integrate traditional healing modalities, such as storytelling, music, art, and dance, into therapeutic interventions.

These cultural practices are not only sources of joy and expression but also serve as powerful tools for healing, self-discovery, and empowerment within the Black community.

Furthermore, the digital age has enabled the expansion of communal healing practices beyond physical spaces, allowing for virtual support groups, online forums, and social media communities that provide a sense of connection and belonging for individuals who may not have access to in-person resources.

Overall, modern adaptations of communal healing practices continue to uphold the values of collectivism, mutual support, and cultural resilience that have long been central to the Black experience.

By fostering a sense of community, belonging, and shared healing, these practices empower individuals to navigate the complexities of modern life while honoring their ancestral traditions and promoting holistic wellbeing.

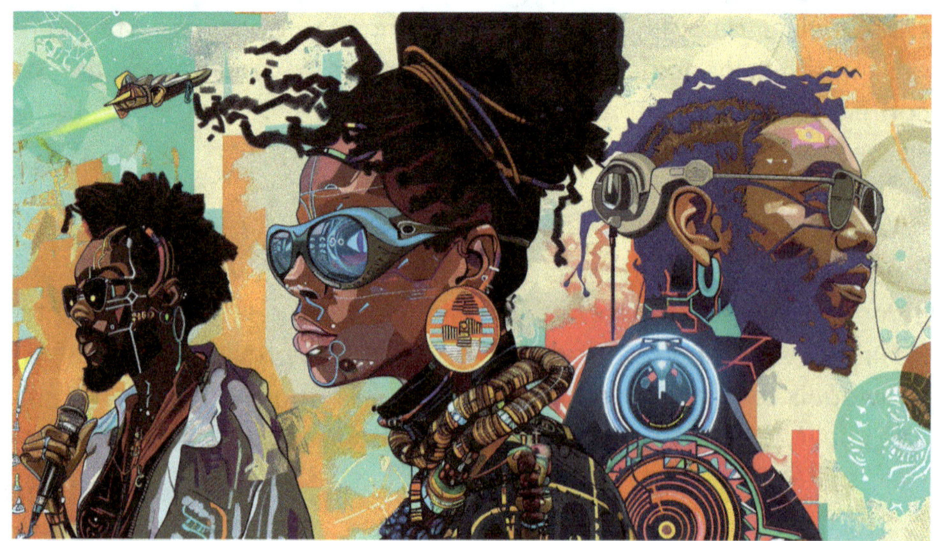

2.4: Building and leveraging support networks for overall wellbeing

Building and leveraging support networks for overall wellbeing is a crucial aspect of holistic wellness in the Black community. Historically, Black individuals have relied on extended family and community connections for emotional, mental, and physical support.

These support networks provide a sense of belonging, understanding, and solidarity that can significantly impact an individual's overall wellbeing.

In the Black experience, the role of extended family and community in mental health is profound. The concept of "it takes a village" is ingrained in many Black cultures, emphasizing the importance of collective care and support.

Extended family members, friends, neighbors, and community organizations play a vital role in providing emotional support, guidance, and practical help during challenging times. This network of support helps individuals navigate life's ups and downs with a sense of security and belonging.

Modern adaptations of communal healing practices have evolved to meet the changing needs of the Black community. While traditional family gatherings and community events remain pillars of support, virtual platforms and social media have also become valuable tools for connecting with others and seeking support.

Online support groups, wellness communities, and mental health resources tailored to the Black experience have emerged as spaces for sharing experiences, seeking advice, and building connections with like-minded individuals.

Building and leveraging support networks for overall wellbeing involves actively seeking out and nurturing relationships that promote positive mental health and holistic wellness.

This may include participating in cultural events, joining community organizations, attending support groups, or connecting with mental health professionals who understand the unique challenges faced by the Black community.

Support networks can also play a crucial role in addressing systemic inequalities and promoting social justice within the Black community. By coming together to advocate for change, support networks can empower individuals to challenge oppressive systems, promote equity and inclusivity, and foster a sense of collective resilience and empowerment.

By drawing on the strength of extended family and community connections, modern adaptations of communal healing practices, and the power of collective action, individuals can cultivate a sense of belonging, resilience, and empowerment that nurtures their physical, emotional, and spiritual health.

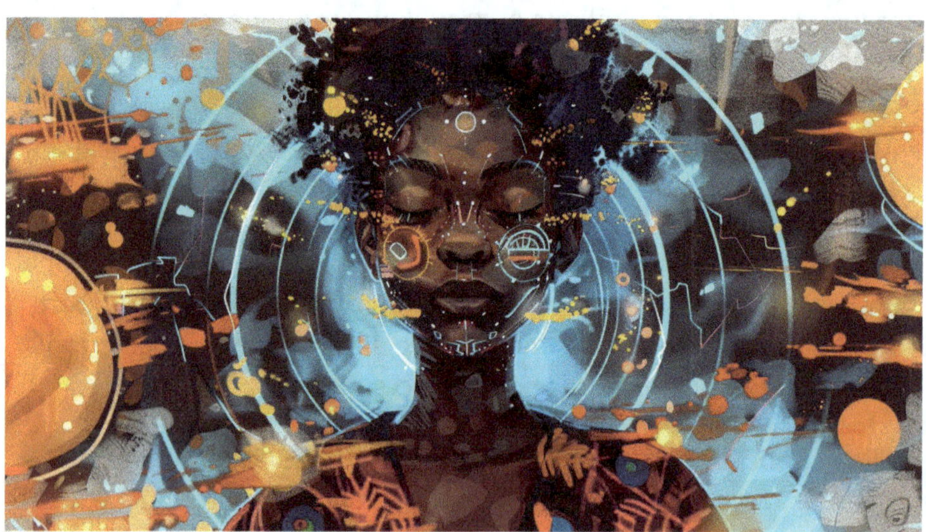

3.1: African dance forms and their health benefits

African dance forms hold a rich cultural significance and are deeply intertwined with physical and spiritual wellness in Black traditions. These traditional movements go beyond mere physical exercise; they embody a holistic approach to health that nurtures the body, mind, and spirit.

African dance forms are not just about choreography; they are about storytelling, community bonding, and connecting with one's roots.

One of the key health benefits of African dance forms is their ability to provide a full-body workout. These dances involve a combination of rhythmic movements, footwork, and body isolations that engage various muscle groups. Unlike conventional exercise routines that focus on repetitive movements,

African dance forms offer a dynamic and expressive way to stay active. The fluidity and energy of these dances promote cardiovascular health, improve flexibility, and enhance coordination.

Moreover, African dance forms are deeply rooted in cultural traditions and spirituality, which adds a unique dimension to their health benefits. The rhythmic drumming, chanting, and storytelling that accompany these dances create a sense of communal connection and shared experience.

This communal aspect of African dance forms fosters a sense of belonging and social support, which are essential for overall well-being and mental health in the Black community.

Another significant health benefit of African dance forms is their ability to promote emotional well-being and stress relief. The expressive nature of these dances allows individuals to release pent-up emotions, express joy and sorrow, and connect with their inner selves.

The cathartic nature of African dance forms can be a powerful tool for managing stress, anxiety, and emotional trauma, providing a safe space for healing and self-expression.

Additionally, African dance forms have been shown to have spiritual and therapeutic benefits. The rhythmic movements and trance-like states induced by these dances can lead to a sense of spiritual connection and transcendence.

Many African dance forms are steeped in spiritual symbolism and ritual, offering practitioners a way to connect with their ancestors, gods, and spiritual guides. This spiritual aspect of African dance forms can provide a sense of purpose, meaning, and inner peace.

Incorporating traditional African dance forms into modern exercise routines can be a transformative experience that nourishes the body, mind, and spirit.

By embracing these cultural practices, individuals can tap into a rich heritage of movement, music, and storytelling that promotes physical fitness, emotional well-being, and spiritual growth. African dance forms offer a holistic approach to health that celebrates diversity, resilience, and the power of community in promoting wellness.

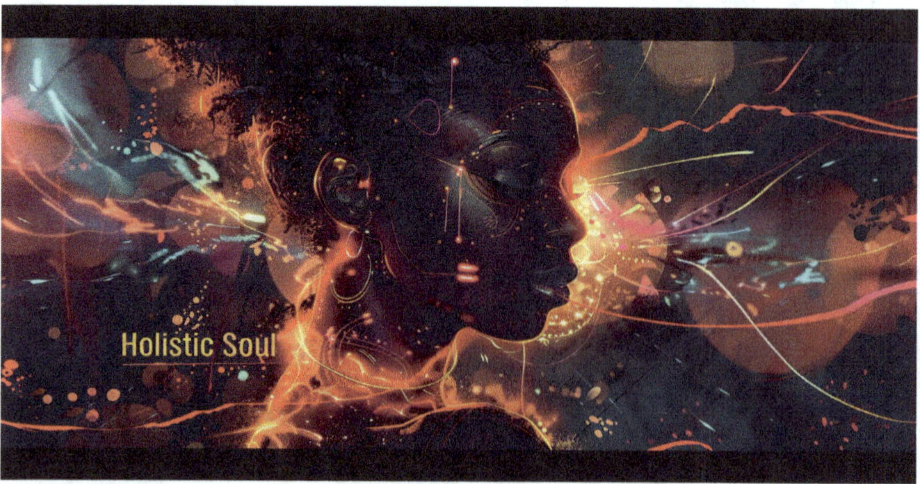

3.2: Incorporating traditional movements into modern exercise routines

Incorporating traditional movements into modern exercise routines offers a unique approach to physical fitness that not only benefits the body but also honors the rich cultural heritage of African and African American communities.

Drawing inspiration from traditional African dance forms and movement practices, this fusion of old and new creates a dynamic and engaging way to stay active and healthy.

African dance forms such as the energetic and rhythmic movements of Afrobeat, the graceful and fluid motions of ballet-inspired African dance, and the powerful and expressive styles of traditional West African dances like the Kpanlogo and Azonto, are not only aesthetically captivating but also provide a full-body workout that strengthens muscles, improves cardiovascular health, and enhances flexibility.

By integrating these traditional movements into modern exercise routines, individuals can experience a holistic approach to fitness that goes beyond just physical benefits. The spiritual and cultural significance of these dances adds an element of mindfulness and connection to one's heritage, fostering a sense of pride and identity that can be empowering and uplifting.

Incorporating traditional African movements into modern exercise routines also offers a fun and engaging way to break away from the monotony of traditional gym workouts.

The infectious rhythms and lively beats of African music can make working out feel more like a celebration than a chore, motivating individuals to stay consistent and committed to their fitness goals.

Moreover, these movements are often designed to be inclusive and accessible to people of all ages and fitness levels, making them ideal for those looking for a low-impact but effective form of exercise.

Whether it's the gentle swaying of hips in a traditional Caribbean dance or the high-energy footwork of South African gumboot dancing, there is a style of African movement for everyone to enjoy.

Incorporating traditional movements into modern exercise routines not only benefits the individual but also contributes to the preservation and celebration of African cultural heritage.

By embracing these practices, individuals can connect with their roots, honor their ancestors, and pass down these valuable traditions to future generations.

By combining the physical benefits of these movements with the spiritual and cultural significance they hold, individuals can achieve a deeper sense of connection, joy, and wellbeing in their fitness journey.

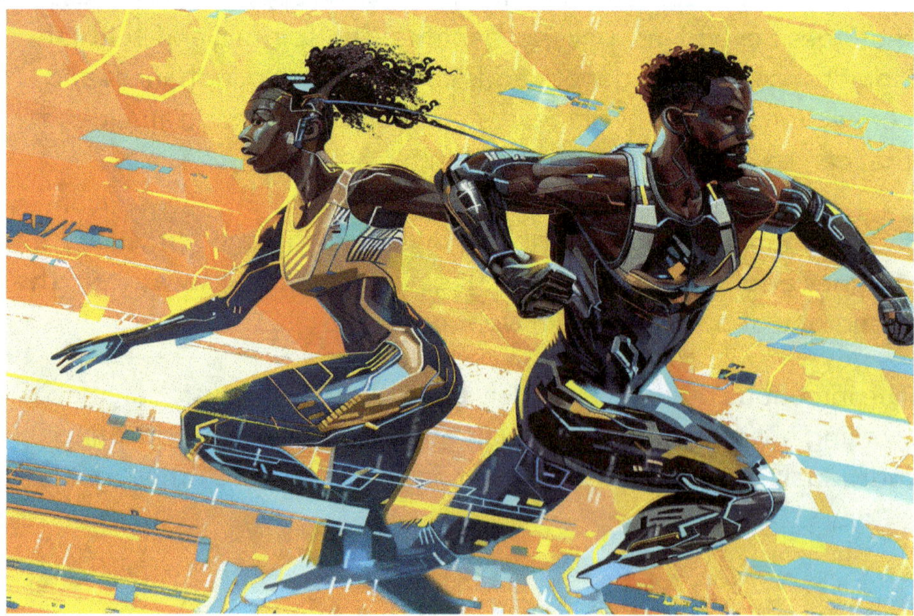

3.3: The spiritual and physical connection in movement practices

The spiritual and physical connection in movement practices is a deeply rooted aspect of African and African American wellness traditions. Movement has been a central component of spiritual and physical well-being in these cultures for generations.

From traditional African dance forms to modern exercise routines, the connection between movement, spirituality, and health is profound and holistic.

African dance forms have long been recognized for their health benefits, both physical and spiritual. These dances are often seen as a form of storytelling, a way to connect with ancestors, and a means of expressing cultural identity.

The movements are not just about physical exercise but also serve as a way to release emotions, heal trauma, and connect with a higher power. African dance is known for its rhythmic and energetic movements that engage the entire body, promoting strength, flexibility, and cardiovascular health.

Incorporating traditional movements into modern exercise routines is a way to honor and preserve cultural heritage while reaping the physical benefits of these practices. By blending traditional African dance moves with contemporary fitness techniques, individuals can experience a unique and enriching workout that not only strengthens the body but also uplifts the spirit.

This fusion of old and new creates a powerful synergy that transcends mere physical fitness and delves into the realm of spiritual well-being.

The spiritual and physical connection in movement practices goes beyond just the movements themselves. It encompasses the intention behind the movement, the mindfulness with which it is performed, and the connection to the broader community.

Movement is seen as a form of prayer, a way to communicate with the divine, and a means of connecting with one's inner self. In African and African American cultures, movement is viewed as a sacred act that can bring about healing, transformation, and unity.

The physical benefits of movement practices are well-documented, with research showing that regular exercise can improve cardiovascular health, boost mood, reduce stress, and increase overall well-being.

When movement is infused with a spiritual intention, it can become a powerful tool for personal growth and self-discovery. By engaging in movement practices that are rooted in a spiritual tradition, individuals can cultivate a deeper connection to their bodies, minds, and spirits.

By honoring and preserving these cultural practices, individuals can experience a holistic approach to health that nurtures the body, mind, and spirit.

Movement is not just about exercise; it is a form of expression, connection, and healing that can transform lives and communities. Embracing the spiritual dimension of movement practices can lead to greater well-being, inner peace, and a deeper sense of connection to oneself and the world around us.

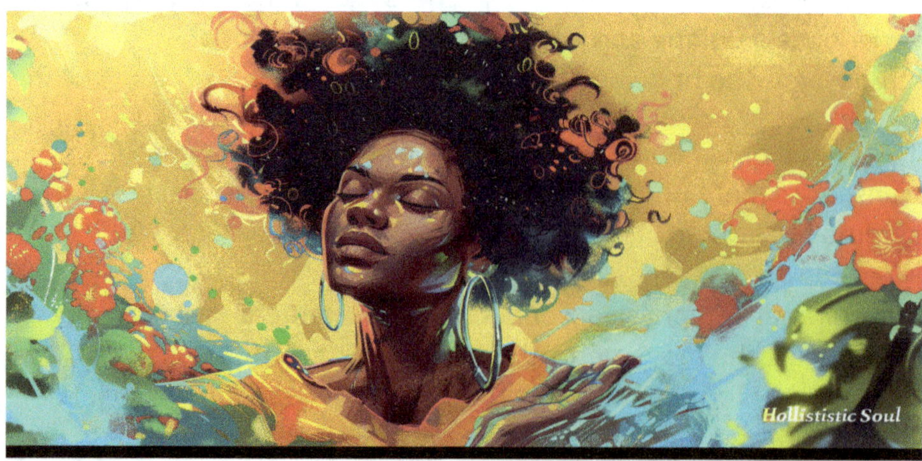

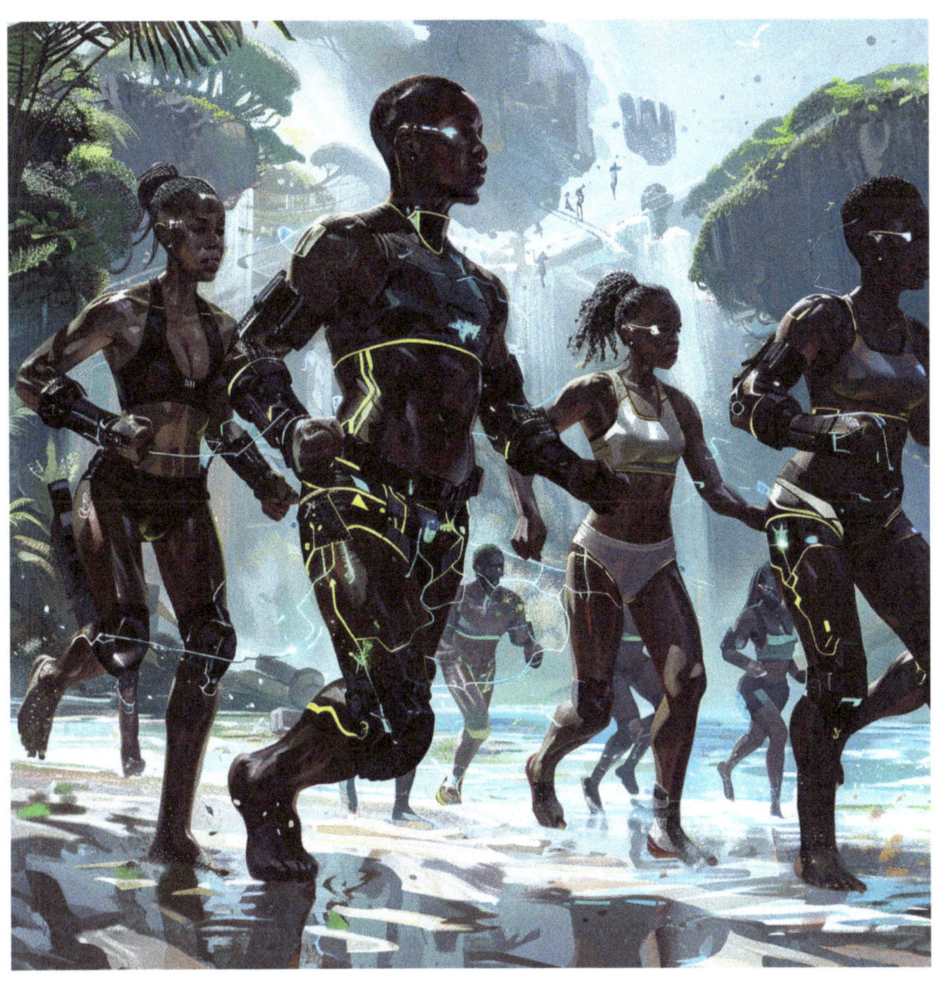

4

Traditional African herbal remedies

Traditional African herbal remedies have been used for centuries to treat various ailments and promote overall well-being. These remedies are deeply rooted in the rich cultural heritage of African communities and are often passed down through generations.

What makes these herbal remedies truly fascinating is that many of them have been found to have scientific backing, showcasing their effectiveness in promoting health and healing.

One of the key aspects of traditional African herbal remedies is the use of medicinal plants that are native to the continent. These plants are often rich in bioactive compounds that have been shown to have therapeutic properties.

For example, plants like African ginger, neem, and moringa have been used for their anti-inflammatory, antimicrobial, and antioxidant properties. Scientific studies have confirmed the efficacy of these plants in treating various conditions such as inflammation, infections, and oxidative stress.

Another important aspect of traditional African herbal remedies is the holistic approach to health and healing. In many African cultures, the concept of wellness is not just limited to the physical body but also encompasses the mind and spirit.

Herbal remedies are often used to restore balance and harmony within the body, promoting overall health and well-being. For example, herbs like African basil and rooibos tea are known for their calming and mood-enhancing effects, making them valuable allies in managing stress and promoting mental health. Moreover, traditional African herbal remedies often take into account the individual's unique constitution and health needs.

Herbalists and healers in African communities are skilled at identifying the root causes of illness and tailoring remedies to address these underlying issues. This personalized approach to healing has been validated by scientific research, which has shown that certain herbal remedies can have specific effects on different body systems based on individual needs.

In addition to their therapeutic properties, traditional African herbal remedies also play a crucial role in preserving biodiversity and supporting sustainable practices. Many of the plants used in these remedies are wildcrafted or grown using traditional farming methods that are environmentally friendly.

By promoting the use of indigenous plants, these remedies help to conserve valuable plant species and protect natural ecosystems.

Overall, traditional African herbal remedies offer a wealth of healing potential that is backed by both cultural wisdom and scientific evidence. By tapping into the knowledge passed down through generations, we can learn valuable lessons about the power of nature to heal and nourish the body, mind, and spirit.

Incorporating these remedies into modern healthcare practices can help us embrace a more holistic approach to wellness that honors our ancestral traditions and promotes optimal health for all.

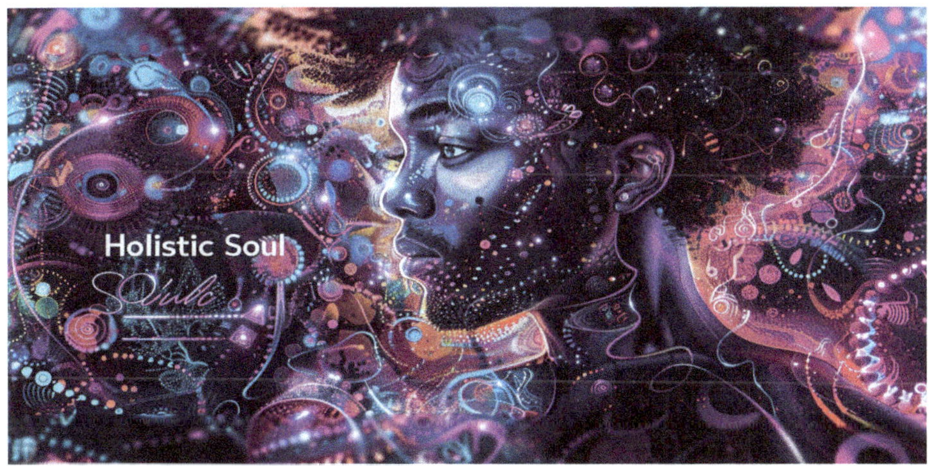

4.2: Slave garden traditions and their modern applications

The practice of cultivating gardens was deeply ingrained in the lives of enslaved Africans brought to the Americas. Despite the harsh conditions they faced, many enslaved individuals maintained small plots of land where they grew their own food. These gardens not only provided sustenance but also served as a form of resistance and a source of autonomy in the face of oppression.

Slave garden traditions were rooted in a deep connection to the land and a rich understanding of plant medicine. Enslaved Africans brought with them a wealth of knowledge about indigenous plants and herbs from their homelands, which they incorporated into their garden practices. These plants were not only used for sustenance but also for healing and spiritual purposes.

Today, we can draw inspiration from these traditions and apply them in modern contexts to promote health and well-being. One way to do this is by growing traditional African crops and herbs in our own gardens. Many of these plants, such as okra, black-eyed peas, and collard greens, are not only delicious but also highly nutritious, rich in vitamins, minerals, and antioxidants.

Incorporating these traditional crops into our diets can help us reconnect with our culinary heritage and benefit from the health-promoting properties of these foods. For example, okra is known for its high fiber content and potential blood sugar-lowering effects, while collard greens are a good source of vitamins A, C, and K.

Furthermore, many of the herbs used in traditional African medicine have been scientifically proven to have medicinal properties. For instance, hibiscus tea, a popular beverage in many African cultures, has been shown to have antioxidant and anti-inflammatory effects. By growing and using these herbs in our own gardens, we can tap into their healing potential and incorporate them into our wellness routines.

Another way to honor slave garden traditions is by creating community gardens that serve as spaces for healing and connection. By coming together to cultivate and harvest food, we can foster a sense of community and shared purpose.

This collective effort not only promotes physical health through access to fresh produce but also supports mental and emotional well-being through social connection.

By growing traditional crops and herbs, creating community gardens, and honoring the knowledge of our ancestors, we can reclaim our culinary heritage, connect with the land, and nurture our bodies and spirits. Through these practices, we can pay homage to the resilience and ingenuity of enslaved Africans while cultivating a sense of empowerment and healing in our own lives.

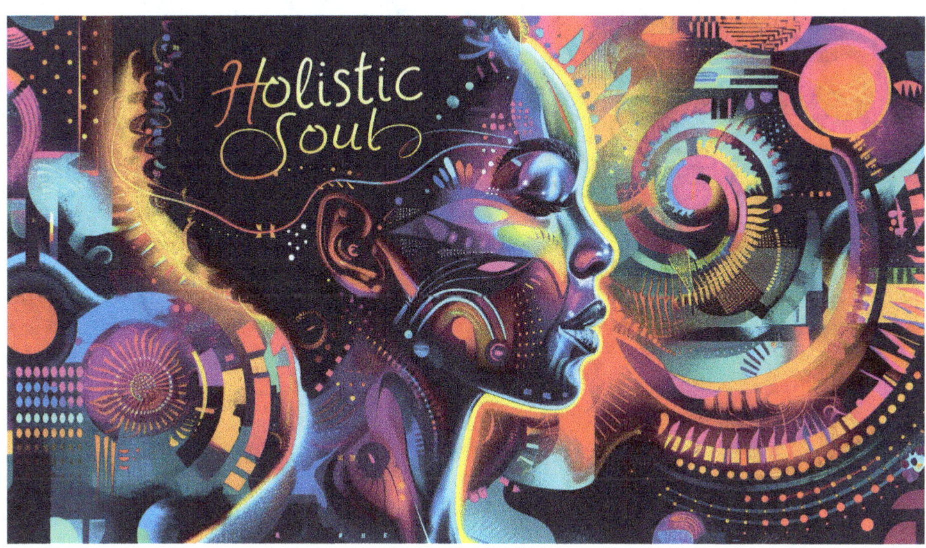

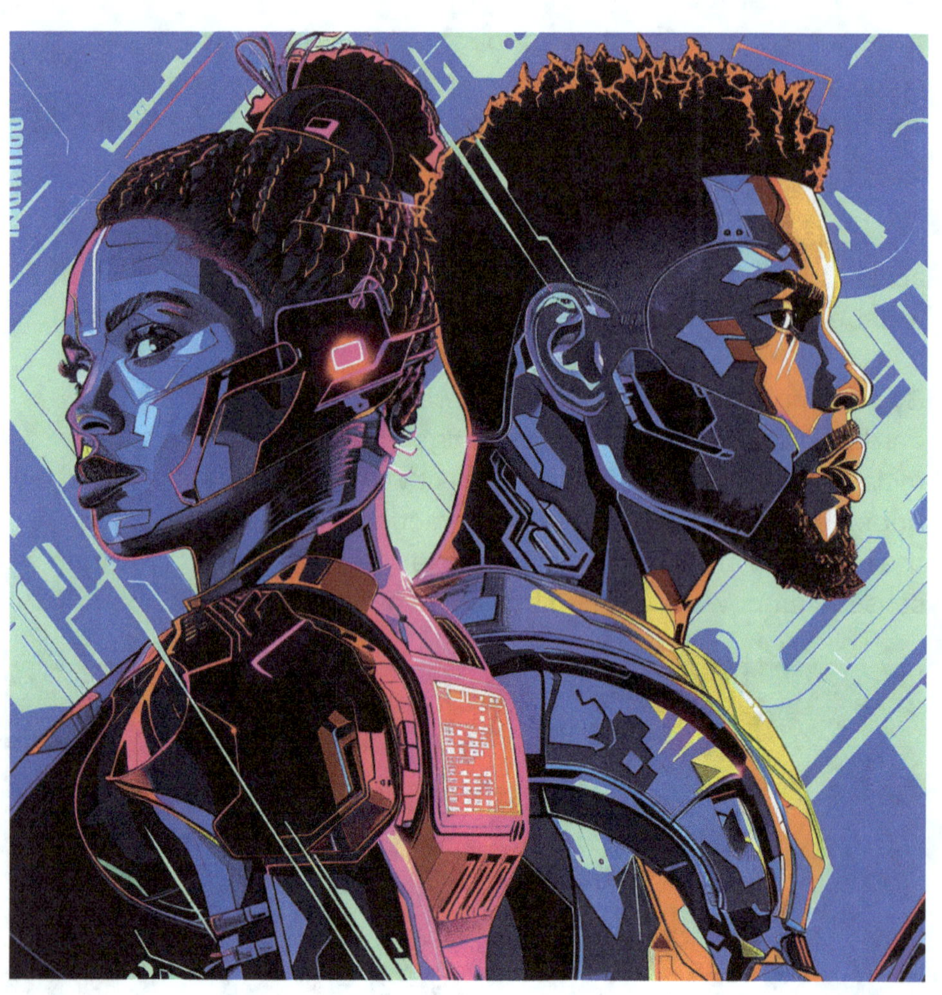

4.3: Integrating herbal treatments with conventional medicine

Integrating herbal treatments with conventional medicine is a practice that has been rooted deeply in African traditions for centuries. Traditional African herbal remedies have been used to treat various ailments and promote overall well-being.

In recent times, there has been a resurgence of interest in these natural remedies as people seek alternative and complementary approaches to conventional medicine.

One of the key aspects of integrating herbal treatments with conventional medicine is understanding the science behind these traditional remedies. Many African herbs have been studied and shown to possess medicinal properties that can complement modern medical treatments.

For example, plants like turmeric, moringa, and African ginger have anti-inflammatory and antioxidant properties that can aid in managing conditions such as arthritis, diabetes, and heart disease.

Furthermore, herbal remedies can also be used to support the body's natural healing processes and boost the immune system. Plants like echinacea, elderberry, and soursop have been traditionally used to strengthen the immune system and fight off infections.

Integrating these herbs into one's daily routine can help prevent illness and support overall health.

Another important aspect of integrating herbal treatments with conventional medicine is ensuring proper dosages and avoiding interactions with prescription medications. It is essential to consult with a healthcare provider or herbalist before incorporating herbal remedies into your healthcare regimen, especially if you are currently taking medications.

Herbal supplements can sometimes interact with prescription drugs, affecting their efficacy or causing adverse effects.

Moreover, integrating herbal treatments with conventional medicine involves understanding the holistic approach to health and wellness. Traditional African healing practices view the body, mind, and spirit as interconnected, and herbal remedies are often used to address imbalances in these areas.

For example, herbs like ashwagandha and valerian root can be used to promote relaxation and improve sleep quality, which can have a positive impact on mental health. By understanding the science behind traditional African herbal remedies, consulting with healthcare providers, and adopting a holistic view of health, individuals can benefit from the synergistic effects of combining natural remedies with modern medical treatments.

This integrative approach can help promote overall well-being and support the body's innate ability to heal itself.

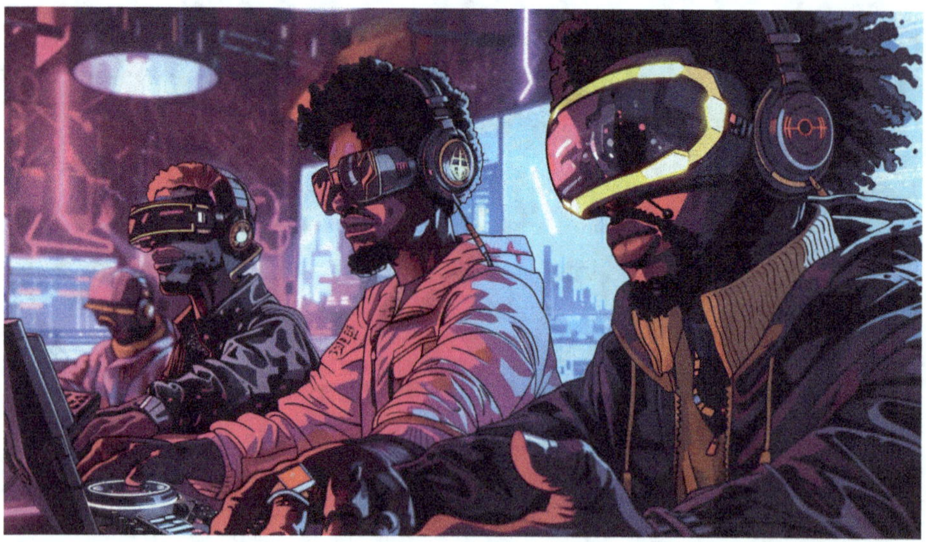

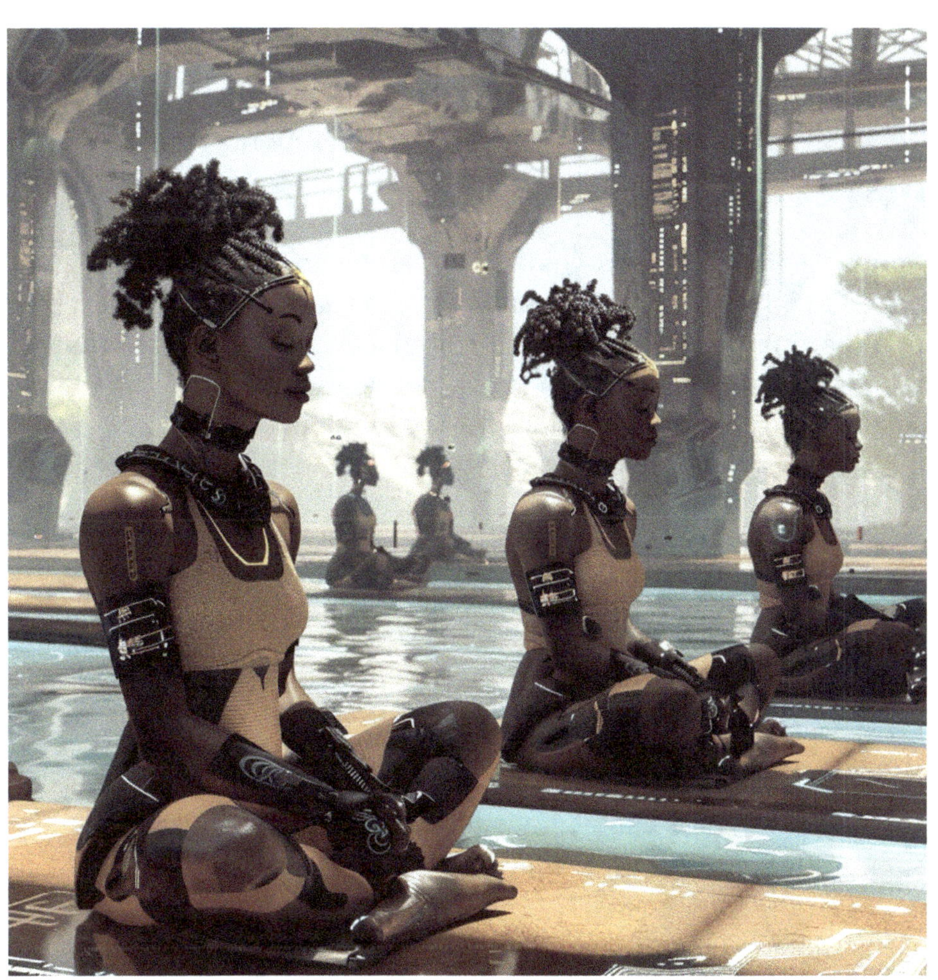

5

The role of spirituality in African and African American healing practices

Spirituality has always been deeply intertwined with healing practices in African and African American traditions. It is believed that the connection between the spiritual and physical realms plays a significant role in maintaining overall wellness and balance. In this section, we will explore the importance of spirituality in healing practices within these communities.

One of the key aspects of spirituality in African and African American healing practices is the belief in the interconnectedness of all things. This interconnectedness is often expressed through rituals, ceremonies, and prayers that honor ancestors, nature, and the divine.

By recognizing and honoring this interconnectedness, individuals are able to tap into a source of strength and guidance that can support them in times of need.

Meditation and mindfulness techniques are also integral parts of spiritual healing practices in these communities. These practices are often rooted in ancient traditions and are used to quiet the mind, center oneself, and connect with the spiritual realm.

Through meditation and mindfulness, individuals are able to cultivate a sense of inner peace, clarity, and purpose, which can have a profound impact on their overall well-being.

Balancing traditional spiritual practices with modern mental health approaches is another important aspect of spirituality in African and African American healing practices. While traditional rituals and ceremonies can provide a sense of connection and support, it is also important to recognize the value of modern mental health techniques such as therapy and counseling.

By integrating these approaches, individuals can create a holistic and comprehensive healing plan that addresses both the spiritual and psychological aspects of their well-being.

Spirituality also plays a role in promoting resilience and coping mechanisms within African and African American communities. Through spiritual practices, individuals are able to draw upon a deep well of strength and courage that can help them navigate through life's challenges and hardships.

Whether through prayer, meditation, or community rituals, spirituality serves as a source of comfort and empowerment for many individuals facing adversity.

Overall, the role of spirituality in African and African American healing practices is multifaceted and deeply ingrained in the cultural fabric of these communities.

By embracing and honoring spiritual traditions, individuals are able to access a rich source of wisdom, guidance, and support that can contribute to their overall well-being and resilience.

Through the integration of spiritual practices with modern approaches to mental health and wellness, individuals can cultivate a holistic and balanced approach to healing that honors their cultural heritage and promotes a sense of wholeness and vitality.

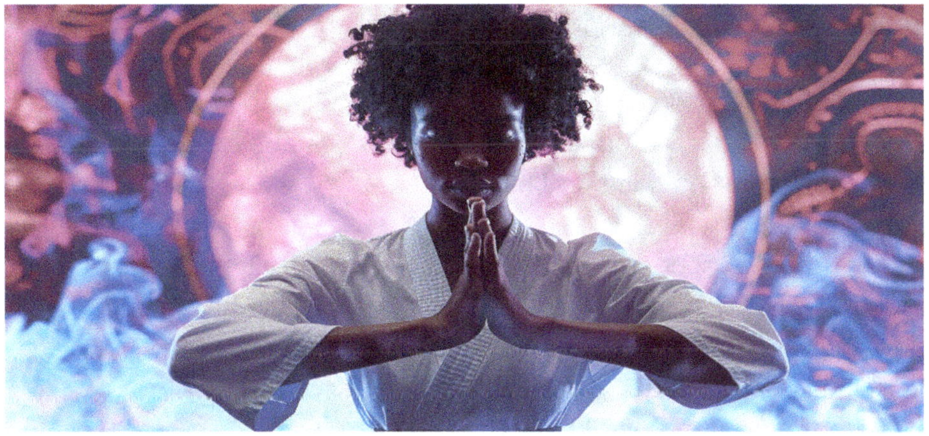

5.2: Meditation and mindfulness techniques rooted in Black traditions

 Meditation and mindfulness are essential components of wellness practices deeply rooted in Black traditions. In African and African American healing practices, the role of spirituality is central to achieving overall wellbeing.

Meditation and mindfulness techniques have been utilized for centuries as tools for inner peace, emotional balance, and spiritual connection.
Within the context of Black traditions, meditation is seen as a practice that allows individuals to connect with their ancestors, the divine, and their inner selves. It is a way to cultivate a sense of grounding and centeredness in the midst of life's challenges and complexities.

Through meditation, individuals can tap into their inner wisdom, find clarity in their thoughts, and cultivate a deeper understanding of their purpose and path in life.

Mindfulness, on the other hand, is about being fully present in the moment, without judgment or attachment to the past or future. In Black traditions, mindfulness is often practiced through various rituals and ceremonies that encourage individuals to be aware of their surroundings, emotions, and thoughts.

By practicing mindfulness, individuals can develop a greater sense of self-awareness, compassion for themselves and others, and an overall sense of balance and harmony.

One of the key aspects of meditation and mindfulness in Black traditions is the emphasis on community and collective healing. In African and African American cultures, the concept of Ubuntu, which means "I am because we are," underscores the interconnectedness of all beings.

Meditation and mindfulness practices are often done in group settings, where individuals come together to support and uplift each other on their healing journeys.

Incorporating meditation and mindfulness into daily life can have profound effects on mental, emotional, and spiritual wellbeing. Studies have shown that regular meditation practice can reduce stress, anxiety, and depression, improve focus and concentration, and enhance overall feelings of peace and contentment.

In Black traditions, meditation and mindfulness techniques are often intertwined with music, dance, and storytelling. Drumming, chanting, and movement are used to enhance the meditative experience and deepen the connection to one's spiritual roots.

By incorporating these elements into meditation practices, individuals can experience a holistic sense of wellness that nurtures the body, mind, and spirit.

 By embracing these ancient practices and integrating them into modern wellness routines, individuals can tap into the wisdom of their ancestors, find peace in the present moment, and cultivate a deep sense of connection to themselves, their community, and the universe at large.

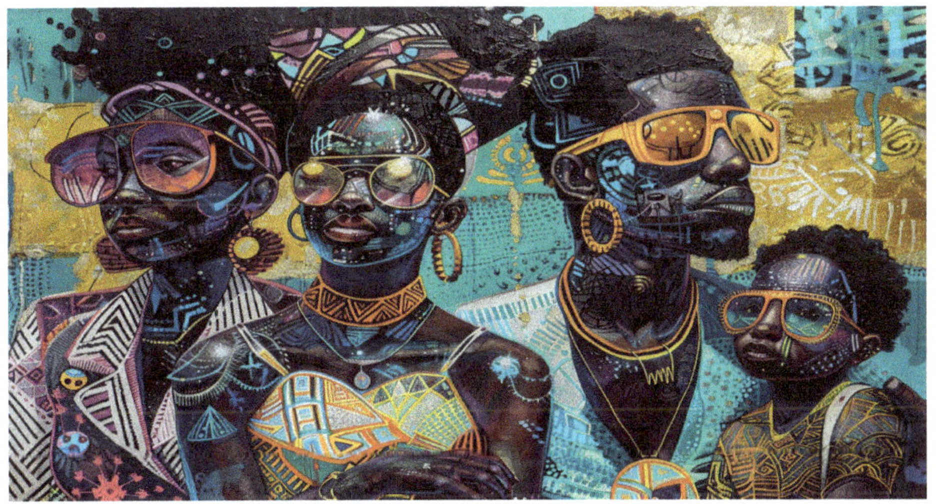

5.3: Balancing traditional spiritual practices with modern mental health approaches

Balancing traditional spiritual practices with modern mental health approaches is a crucial aspect of overall wellness in the Black community. Throughout history, African and African American healing practices have often integrated spirituality as a key component in promoting mental well-being.

This holistic approach recognizes the interconnectedness of the mind, body, and spirit in achieving optimal health.

Spirituality plays a significant role in traditional African and African American cultures, providing a foundation for coping with challenges, finding inner peace, and fostering a sense of community and belonging.

Practices such as prayer, meditation, drumming, chanting, and other rituals are deeply rooted in these cultures and have been passed down through generations as sources of strength and resilience.

In modern mental health approaches, there is a growing recognition of the importance of incorporating spiritual practices into therapy and treatment plans. Research has shown that spirituality can have a positive impact on mental health outcomes, including reducing symptoms of anxiety, depression, and stress. By integrating traditional spiritual practices into therapy sessions, individuals can draw on their cultural heritage to find comfort, guidance, and healing.

Meditation and mindfulness techniques rooted in Black traditions offer powerful tools for managing stress, improving focus, and cultivating a sense of inner peace. Practices such as mindfulness meditation, breathwork, and visualization can help individuals connect with their spiritual beliefs, enhance self-awareness, and promote emotional well-being.

Balancing traditional spiritual practices with modern mental health approaches involves creating a safe and inclusive space where individuals can explore their beliefs, values, and cultural heritage in the context of their mental health journey.

Therapists and mental health professionals who are culturally competent and aware of the significance of spirituality in the lives of their clients can provide a more holistic and effective approach to treatment.

It is essential to recognize the diversity of spiritual beliefs and practices within the Black community and to respect each individual's unique relationship with spirituality.

By honoring and integrating traditional spiritual practices into mental health care, individuals can access a deeper sense of meaning, purpose, and connection that can support their healing and growth.

In conclusion, balancing traditional spiritual practices with modern mental health approaches is a dynamic process that empowers individuals to draw on the wisdom of their ancestors while embracing contemporary therapeutic interventions.

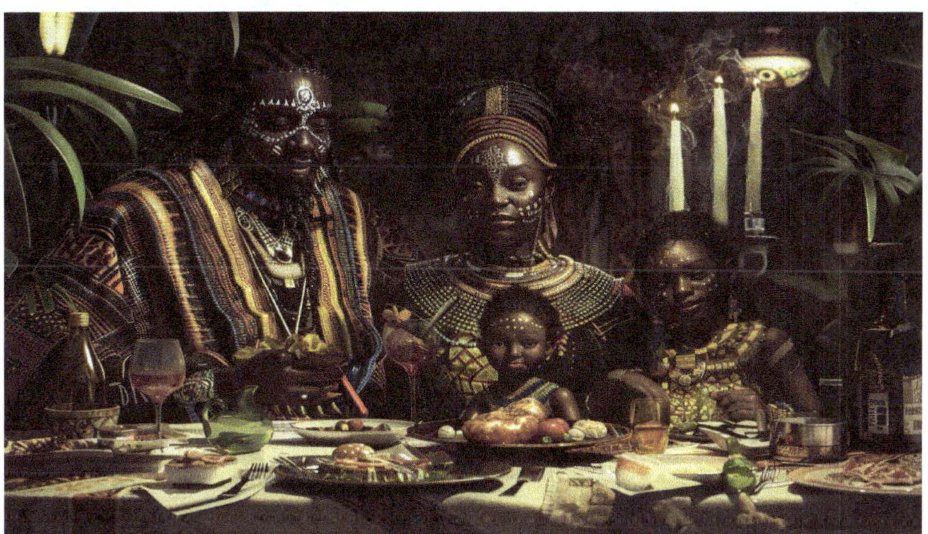

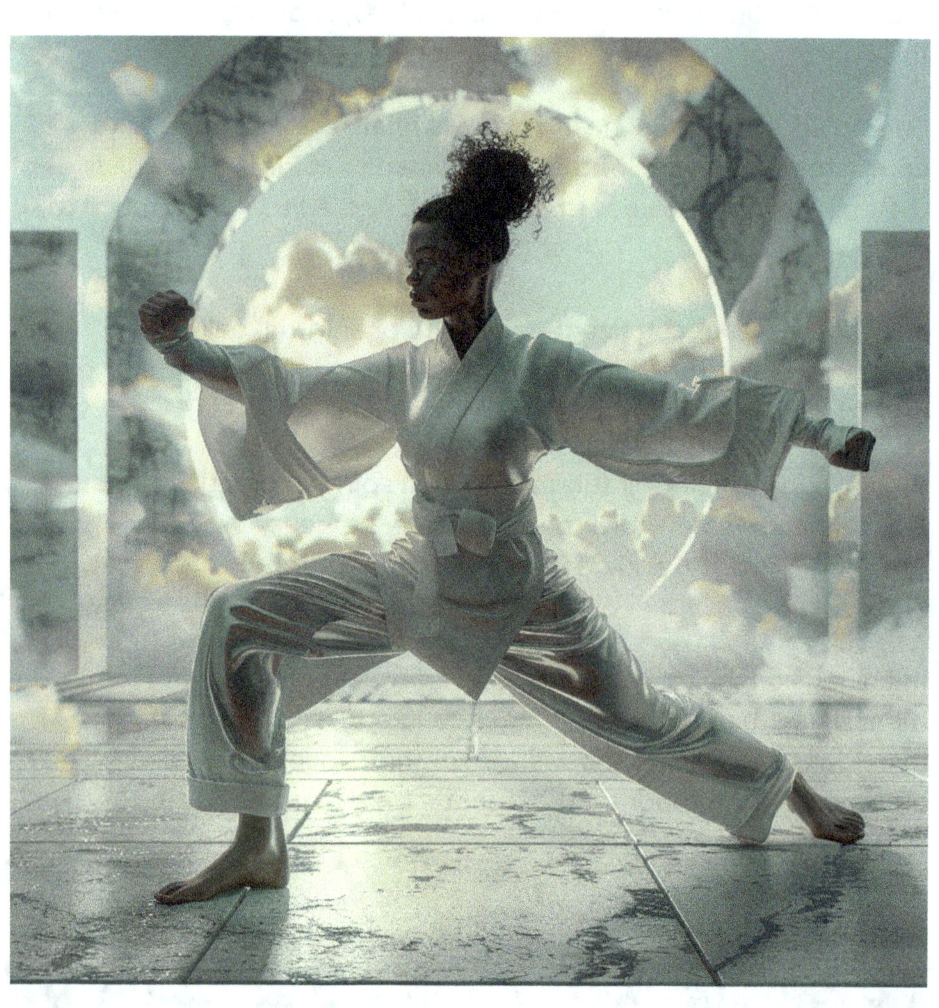

6

Traditional African beauty and skincare practices

Traditional African beauty and skincare practices are deeply rooted in history and cultural traditions that have been passed down through generations. These practices not only focus on enhancing physical appearance but also prioritize overall wellness and self-care. From ancient times to modern-day,

African communities have valued natural ingredients and holistic approaches to skincare that promote health from the inside out.

One key aspect of Traditional African beauty and skincare practices is the use of natural ingredients sourced from the environment. African botanicals such as shea butter, coconut oil, baobab oil, and African black soap are commonly used in skincare routines for their nourishing and healing properties.

These ingredients are rich in vitamins, minerals, and antioxidants that help to hydrate, protect, and rejuvenate the skin. They are often combined with local herbs and plant extracts known for their anti-inflammatory and antibacterial properties, such as aloe vera, neem, and moringa.

In addition to using natural ingredients, Traditional African beauty and skincare practices also emphasize the importance of rituals and self-care routines. Cleansing, exfoliating, and moisturizing are essential steps in maintaining healthy skin, and African traditions often involve elaborate rituals that incorporate massage, aromatherapy, and spiritual elements.

For example, traditional African women may use facial steaming with herbs like eucalyptus or rosemary to purify the skin and promote relaxation. Furthermore, Traditional African beauty and skincare practices recognize the interconnectedness of the body, mind, and spirit.

Beauty rituals are seen as a way to honor one's body and maintain a harmonious balance between inner and outer beauty. This holistic approach to skincare emphasizes the importance of self-love, self-acceptance, and self-expression, encouraging individuals to embrace their natural beauty and uniqueness.

Another important aspect of Traditional African beauty and skincare practices is the emphasis on community and intergenerational knowledge sharing. Beauty rituals are often passed down from mothers to daughters, grandmothers to granddaughters, creating a sense of cultural continuity and belonging.

These practices foster a sense of connection to one's heritage and identity, reinforcing the idea that beauty is not just about physical appearance but also about cultural pride and self-expression.

By incorporating natural ingredients, rituals, and a sense of community, these practices promote overall wellness and self-love. Embracing these traditions can not only enhance one's physical appearance but also nurture the soul and spirit, creating a deeper sense of connection to oneself and to the rich cultural heritage of Africa.

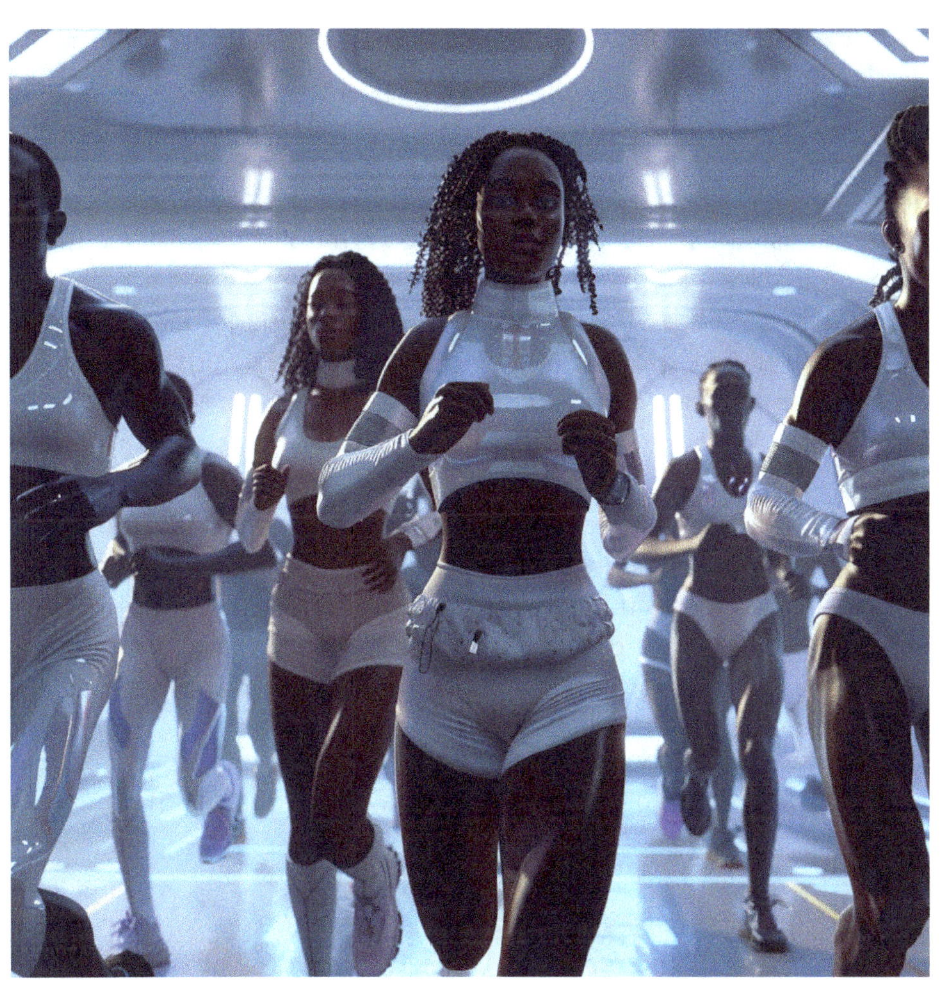

6.2: Stress management techniques drawn from Black cultural wisdom

Stress management techniques drawn from Black cultural wisdom are deeply rooted in traditions that have been passed down through generations. These techniques encompass a holistic approach to managing stress, addressing both the physical and mental aspects of well-being. In the Black community, stress management is viewed as an essential component of maintaining overall health and resilience in the face of adversity.

One key aspect of stress management in Black cultural wisdom is the emphasis on self-care practices that nurture the body and mind. This includes engaging in activities that promote relaxation and rejuvenation, such as taking warm baths infused with herbs or essential oils, practicing meditation and deep breathing exercises, and engaging in physical activities like dancing or walking in nature.

These practices are believed to not only reduce stress levels but also to strengthen the mind-body connection and promote emotional balance.

Another important stress management technique drawn from Black cultural wisdom is the practice of seeking support from community and family. In the Black community, there is a strong tradition of relying on extended family and close-knit social networks for emotional support and guidance.

This sense of community and belonging can provide a sense of security and comfort during times of stress, fostering resilience and emotional well-being.

Additionally, spiritual practices play a significant role in stress management within Black cultural traditions. Many African and African American spiritual practices emphasize the importance of connecting with a higher power or spiritual force for guidance and strength.

Prayer, meditation, and mindfulness techniques rooted in Black traditions can help individuals find inner peace and a sense of calm in the midst of life's challenges.

Furthermore, stress management in Black cultural wisdom often involves incorporating traditional healing practices, such as herbal remedies and natural therapies, into daily routines. Many herbs and plants have been used for centuries in African and African American healing traditions to promote relaxation, reduce anxiety, and support mental well-being.

By integrating these natural remedies into their self-care routines, individuals can harness the healing power of nature to combat stress and promote overall health.

 Overall, stress management techniques drawn from Black cultural wisdom offer a rich and diverse array of tools for promoting emotional well-being and resilience. By embracing these traditional practices and integrating them into daily life, individuals can cultivate a sense of balance, strength, and inner peace that can help them navigate life's challenges with grace and resilience.

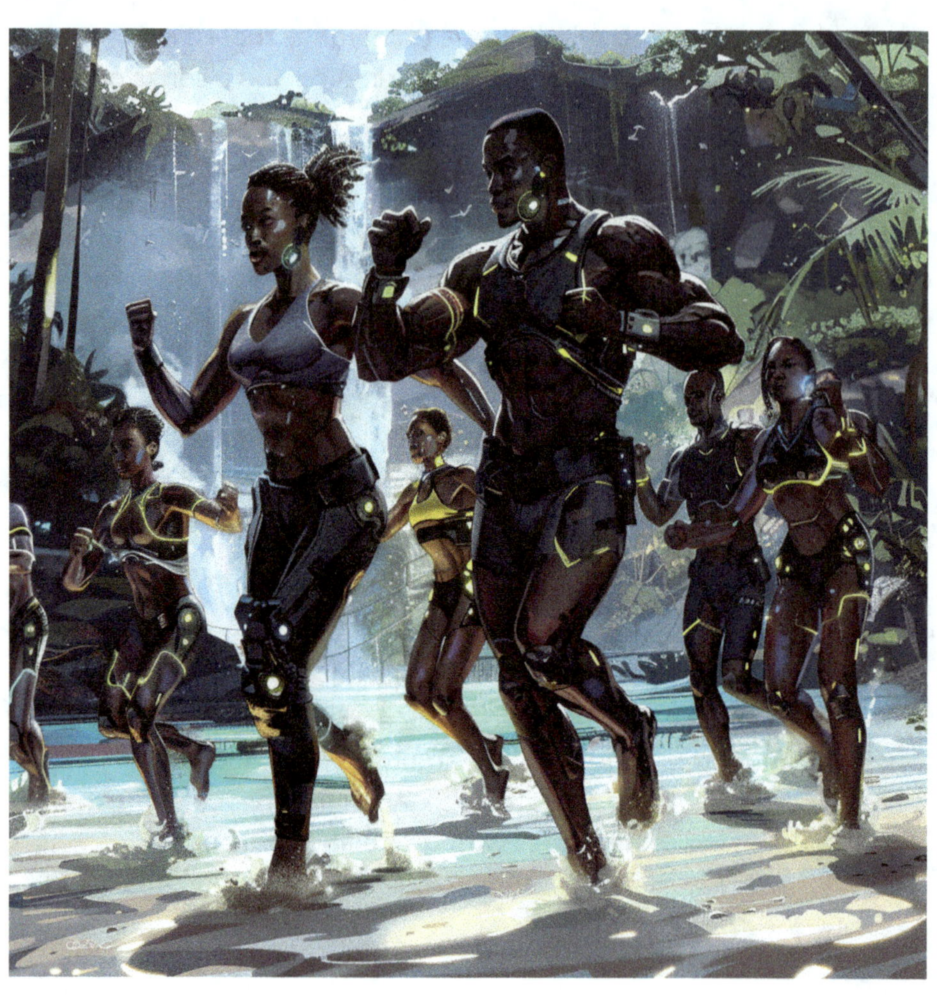

6.3: Sleep and rest practices for optimal health, inspired by ancestral rhythms

Sleep and rest practices for optimal health, inspired by ancestral rhythms, delve deep into the wisdom of traditional African cultures that recognized the importance of rest and rejuvenation for overall well being. The ancient practices of our ancestors provide valuable insights into establishing healthy sleep patterns and optimizing rest for physical, mental, and spiritual wellness.

In traditional African cultures, sleep was considered a sacred time for rejuvenation and spiritual connection. Ancestral rhythms guided daily routines, aligning with the natural cycles of day and night. These rhythms were deeply rooted in the understanding that rest is essential for maintaining balance and harmony within the body and mind.

One key aspect of ancestral sleep practices is the concept of early to bed, early to rise. Our ancestors understood the importance of going to bed at a consistent time each night and waking up with the sunrise.

This practice not only aligns with our natural circadian rhythms but also allows for restorative sleep that enhances physical health and mental clarity.

Another important element of ancestral sleep practices is creating a conducive sleep environment. Traditional African cultures often used natural materials such as cotton and linen for bedding, promoting comfort and breathability during sleep.

Additionally, incorporating calming rituals before bed, such as herbal teas or meditation, can help prepare the mind and body for restful sleep. Furthermore, ancestral rhythms emphasize the importance of honoring the body's need for rest and relaxation. In modern society, we often prioritize productivity over rest, leading to chronic stress and sleep deprivation.

By drawing inspiration from ancestral practices, we can cultivate a mindset that values rest as a vital component of self-care and overall health.

Ancestral sleep practices also highlight the significance of establishing bedtime rituals that signal the body to unwind and prepare for sleep. This could include activities such as gentle stretching, journaling, or listening to soothing music.

By incorporating these rituals into our nightly routine, we can create a sense of calm and relaxation that promotes restful sleep.

Moreover, ancestral wisdom teaches us to listen to our bodies and honor our individual sleep needs. Just as our ancestors recognized the importance of restorative sleep, we too can benefit from tuning into our natural rhythms and adjusting our sleep habits accordingly.

In conclusion, sleep and rest practices inspired by ancestral rhythms offer valuable insights into cultivating optimal health and wellbeing. By embracing the wisdom of our ancestors and incorporating their teachings into our modern lives, we can enhance our sleep quality, reduce stress, and nurture our bodies and minds for overall wellness.

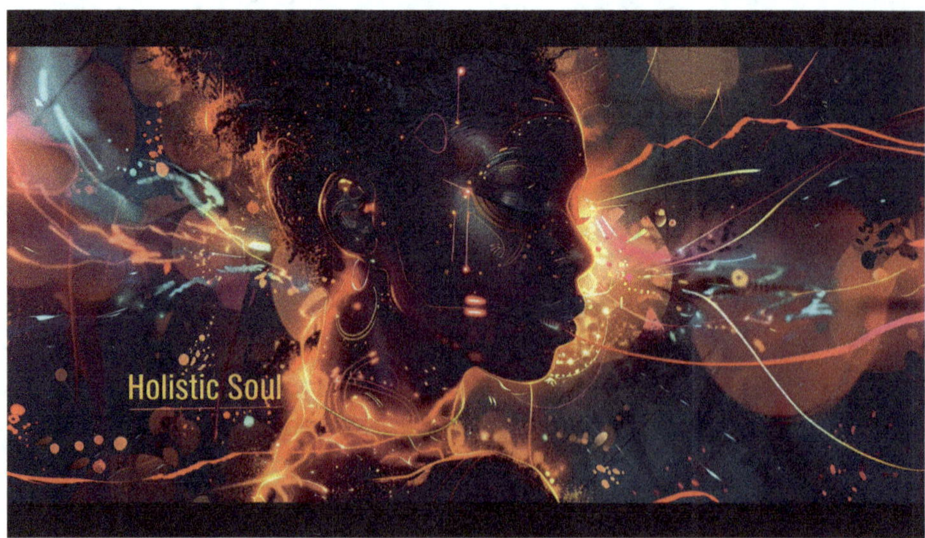

Afterword

Dear Readers,

Thank you from the bottom of my heart for taking the time to read "The Holistic Soul". Your support and engagement mean the world to me.

I hope this book has provided you with valuable insights and perhaps a new perspective on holistic well-being. My goal was to create a resource that could guide you on your journey towards a more balanced and fulfilling life.

Your decision to invest your time and energy in this book is deeply appreciated. I believe that every reader brings their own unique experiences to the text, enriching its meaning in countless ways.

If "The Holistic Soul" has touched your life in any way, I'd be honored to hear about it. Your stories and feedback not only inspire me but also help to create a community of like-minded individuals on the path to holistic health.

Thank you again for being a part of this journey. May you continue to nurture your holistic soul and find harmony in all aspects of your life.

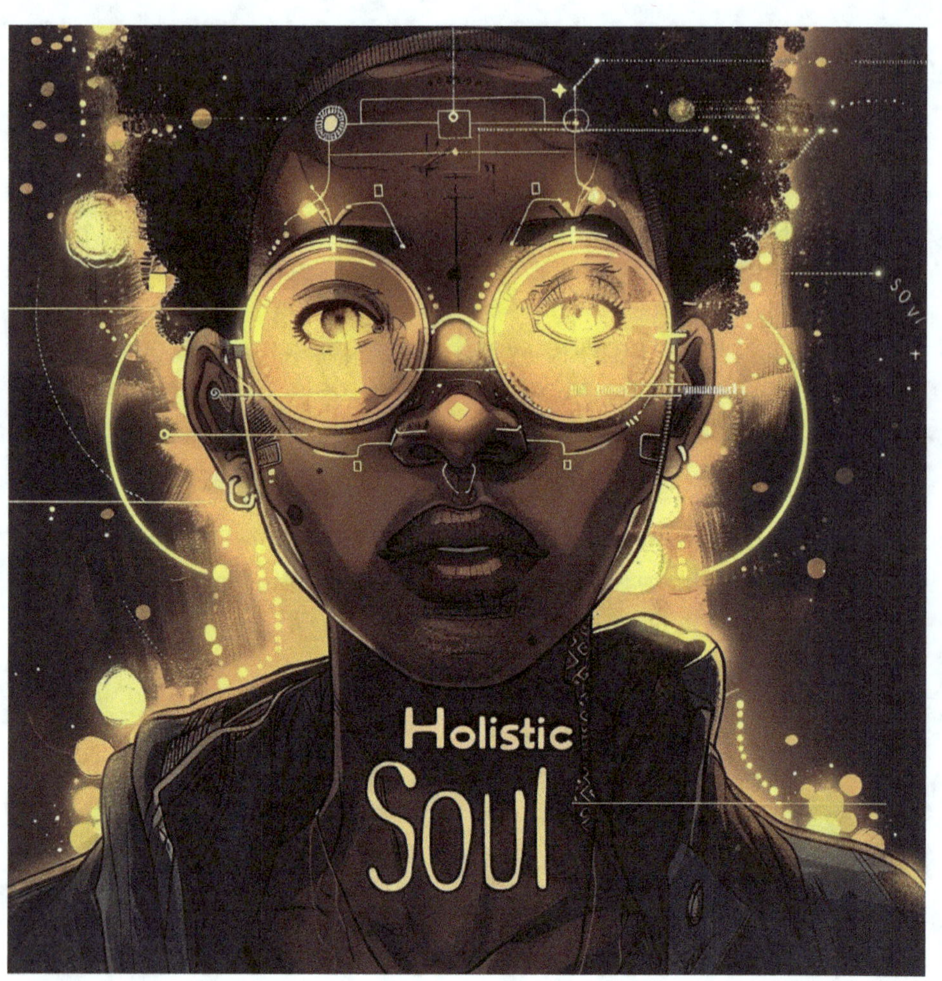
Holistic
Soul

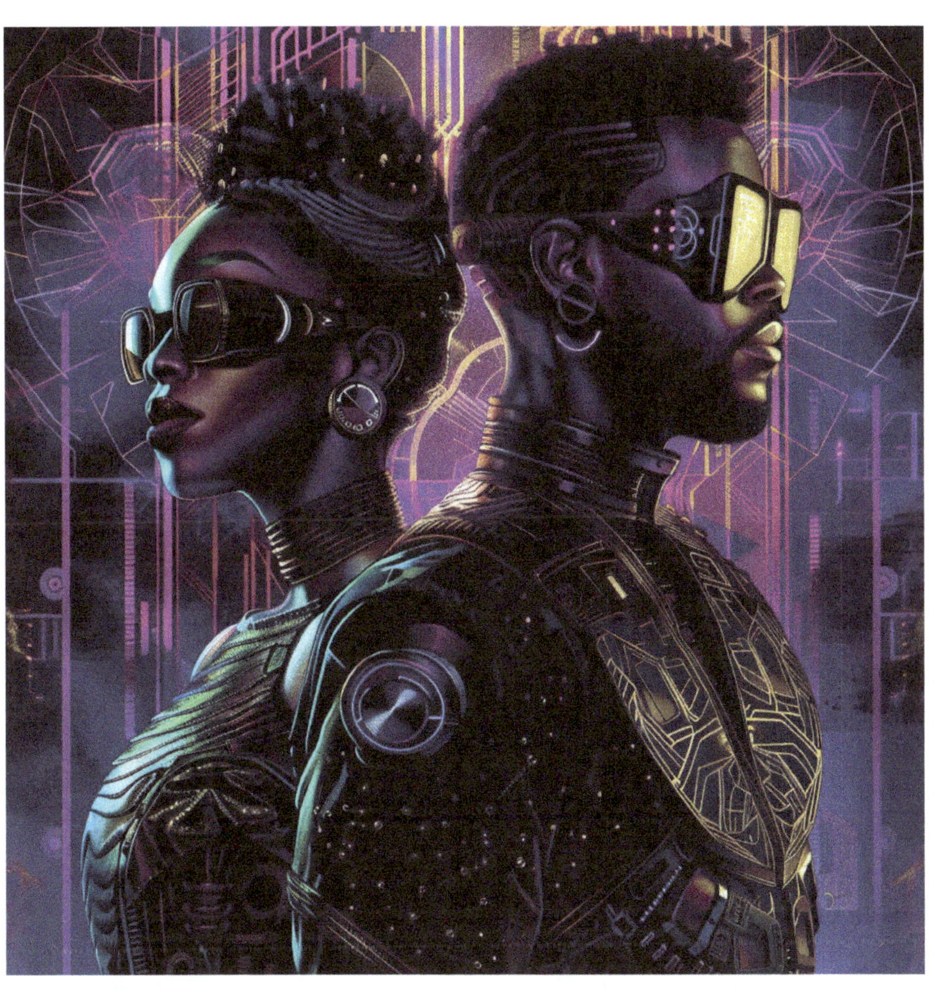

Conclusion:

As we close the pages of "The Holistic Soul: Wellness Practices Rooted in Black Tradition," we find ourselves at the intersection of past and present, tradition and innovation. This journey through the rich landscape of Black wellness practices has been more than an exploration of health strategies; it has been a rediscovery of our cultural heritage and a reimagining of our approach to well-being.

Throughout this book, we've delved into the wisdom of our ancestors, uncovering practices that have sustained Black communities for generations. From the nourishing power of soul food reimagined with superfoods, to the healing rhythms of traditional movement, to the strength found in communal bonds, we've seen how our cultural practices offer a holistic path to health that addresses body, mind, and spirit.

But this journey doesn't end here. The true power of these practices lies not just in knowing them, but in living them. As we move forward, let us carry these teachings with us, integrating them into our daily lives and sharing them with our families and communities. Let us approach our health with the same resilience, creativity, and soul that have defined Black culture throughout history.

Remember, wellness is not a destination but a continuous journey. It's about making choices each day that honor our bodies, uplift our spirits, and connect us to our roots. It's about finding joy in nourishing meals, strength in movement, peace in spiritual practices, and healing in community.

As you close this book, I challenge you to become a steward of these traditions. Adapt them to your modern life, share them with the next generation, and continue to seek out the wisdom that resides within our culture. In doing so, you not only improve your own health but contribute to the collective well-being of our community.

"The Holistic Soul" is more than a guide—it's a testament to the enduring power of Black wellness traditions and their relevance in addressing contemporary health challenges. It's a reminder that within our cultural heritage lies the key to not just surviving, but thriving.

As we face the health challenges of the modern world, let us do so with the strength of our ancestors behind us, the support of our community beside us, and the wisdom of our traditions within us. For in nurturing the health of our bodies and the vitality of our spirits, we honor our past and create a healthier, more vibrant future for generations to come.

May your journey towards holistic health be filled with discovery, empowerment, and the deep, restorative power of practices rooted in the rich soil of Black tradition. Here's to the health of your body, the peace of your mind, and the vibrancy of your soul.

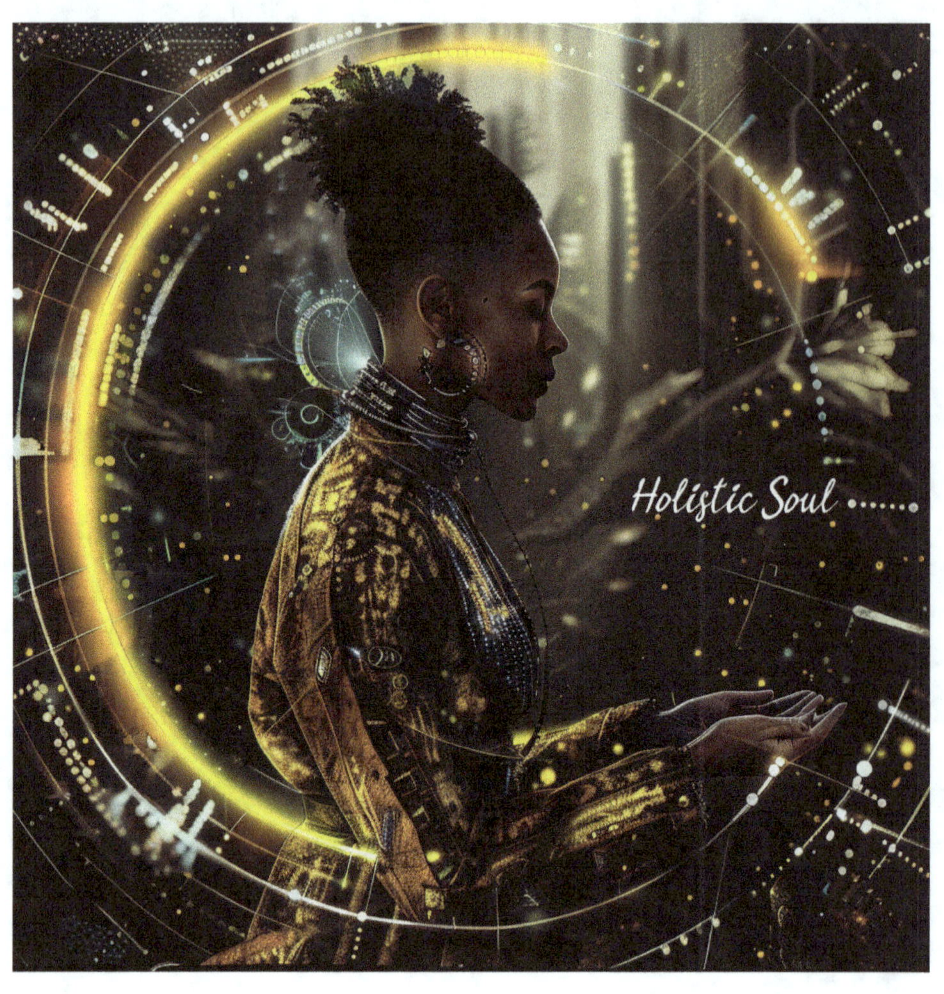

Holistic Soul